Ancient Peoples and Places

THE SCYTHIANS

General Editor

DR GLYN DANIEL

Ancient Peoples and Places

THE SCYTHIANS

Tamara (Abelson) Talbot Rice

63 PHOTOGRAPHS
65 LINE DRAWINGS
AND 4 MAPS

FREDERICK A. PRAEGER *Publisher*
New York

THIS IS VOLUME TWO IN THE SERIES

Ancient Peoples and Places

GENERAL EDITOR: DR. GLYN DANIEL

BOOKS THAT MATTER

Published in the United States of America
in 1957 by Frederick A. Praeger, Inc., Publisher
64 University Place, New York 3, N.Y.
All rights reserved
Library of Congress catalog card number 57-8255

© THAMES AND HUDSON LONDON 1957
SECOND EDITION, 1958
THIRD EDITION, 1961
PRINTED IN GREAT BRITAIN
BY EBENEZER BAYLIS AND SON LTD.
WORCESTER

To those who lived at Volgovo

CONTENTS

ILLUSTRATIONS

The Scythian Kings

TARGITAUS The reputed head of the Phalatæ dynasty, but probably a wholly legendary personage.

COLAXIS Probably founded the dynasty of Royal Scyths.

SPARGAPEITHES

LYCUS Son of Spargapeithes.

GNURUS Son of Lycus.

PARTATUA and his son *Madyes,* possibly his co-ruler or deputy. They ruled in Urartu *c.* 630 B.C.

SAULIUS Brother of Anacharsis, was ruler in 589 B.C.

IDANTHYRSUS With Taxacis and Scopacis (possibly deputies or co-rulers) opposed Darius *c.* 516 B.C.

ARIAPEITHES Son of Idanthyrsus, married a Greek woman from Istrus as well as a Scythian, Opoea, and also the daughter of the Thracian chief Teres.

SCYLES Son of Ariapeithes, at whose death he married his Greek stepmother; killed by his brother Octomasades for his philhellene sympathies.

OCTOMASADAS Succeeded Scyles. Just prior to Herodotus.

ARIANTHAS He held a census of his people.

ARISTAGORAS Reigned *c.* 495 B.C.

ATEAS Killed in battle by Philip of Macedon in 339 B.C. at the age of ninety.

AGARUS Sheltered the youngest son of the Bosphoran ruler Spartocus. The latter was succeeded by his co-ruler Pairisades I, who refused to pay tribute due to the Scythians and was consequently killed in battle by Agarus in 310 B.C.

SCYLURUS Struck coins at Olbia *c.* 110 B.C. and had his capital at Neapolis.

PALAKUS Son of Scylurus.

No man is an island
Entire of itself;
Every man is a piece of the continent
A part of the main.

John Donne

Foreword

I SHOULD LIKE to express my deep appreciation of the ready advice given to me on many occasions by Professor Stuart Piggott, and of the kindness and generosity of Professor Victor Lazarev, of The Art Historical Institute, Moscow, and Dr Alice Bank, of The Hermitage Museum, Leningrad, for their gift of many of the photographs with which this volume is illustrated.

I am likewise very grateful to Professor John Orr for his translation of the quotation from Pushkin; to Mrs Glyn Daniel for the infinite patience with which she worked on the maps illustrating this book; to Dr Davies for checking my list of Asiatic plants; to Mr Leonid Zouroff for telling me a great deal about his researches into the survival of ancient beliefs amongst the Lithuanian peasantry; to Mrs Scott for some excellent drawings; to Miss Timbey of the photographic department or the Society for Cultural Relations with the USSR; to Mr Zarnecki of the Courtauld Institute for helpful advice with regard to illustrations; to Mr. Harold Bowen and Lt./Col. Wheeler for the loan of scarce books; and, above all, to my husband for his unfailing help.

T. T. R.

Introduction

CHANCE, as Conrad liked to call it—luck, or even fate, as others prefer to think—plays its part as much in shaping the destinies of races as of individuals, dispensing vicissitudes or boons alike upon the lone figure and the composite group. Of the vicissitudes the saddest, though assuredly not the most dire, is that by which the dead are relegated to oblivion. It is perhaps a subconscious awareness of this hazard that so often directs the steps of an indolent walker to an old churchyard, leading him to pause by a decayed tombstone, to wonder as he gazes at its perished and illegible inscription as to what manner of man was laid beneath the enigmatic slab, to speculate upon his way of life, and to regret that all traces of this once vital and alert being—even to the record of his name and life span—have now forever faded from the notice of mankind.

Antiquarians are often assailed by somewhat similar thoughts, especially those of them who are attracted by the less well documented pages of ancient history. Amongst the most meagre of such passages, but also amongst the most absorbing, are those dealing with the Scythian nomads, who, in the last millennium of the pre-Christian era, roamed the vast, almost crescent-shaped steppe which stretches from the confines of China to the banks of the Danube. Today, practically the whole immense expanse of natural grassland belongs to the USSR, but in early prehistoric times numerous tribes succeeded each other in this enormous plain. In the north-eastern section many of these peoples often displayed a tendency, which became more marked with the passing centuries, to migrate to the west or south-west of their starting point, a tendency which was doubtless fostered by the existence on their other borders of

B

geographical barriers which debarred them from breaking out in these directions. The trail of their movements can occasion-ally be picked up here and there thanks to the objects they left behind them, but their history is virtually lost to us, even though pre-historians are sometimes able to salvage a few nebulous facts from those ancient, long-forgotten, unrecorded years. A little more information is available about the European section of the steppe during the last millennium of the pre-Christian era; then, the late bronze age inhabitants of the area were succeeded, and eventually assimilated, by tribes whose origins remain obscure, but who, centring round the Royal Scyths of southern Russia, have nevertheless left us numerous, tangible tokens of their existence. Except for their pottery, all of their possessions that have come down to us, including the most utilitarian objects, arrest attention, in part because of the skill with which they were fashioned, in part because of the strongly individual style of the animal representations with which the vast majority are decorated. These figures reveal a preoccupation with the animal world, which is accompanied by the ability to express this world's essential features with a directness, conviction and sumptuousness that have not so far found a parallel in any other school of nomadic art. Indeed, the animal forms which the Scythians created for their own delight are so vital and seductive that they eventually affected the art of much of western Europe, permanently marking it with their own individual stamp.

It is a great pity that the Scythians did not possess an alphabet or a coinage, for although the startling variety of the objects retrieved from their burials testifies to an unexpectedly complex way of life and to an almost universal talent for design, our knowledge of them must largely depend upon secondary sources. First-hand information is limited to the deductions which can be drawn from excavating their tombs, and for basic historical facts we have to turn to the sparse references which their more cultured contemporaries, whether Chinese, Assyrians, Jews or Greeks, happened to make to them in their written records and also to the more detailed, if confused, accounts compiled by Greek historians of the classical age.

Many ancient Greek scholars mistakenly considered the Scythians the world's oldest race. Trogus Pompeius, writing in the first century B.C., affirmed that they had always been thought so by all but the Egyptians, who had long disputed the assertion. In this instance the Egyptians were indeed in the right, for, in contradiction to their own account of their origins, the Scythians did not become a recognizable national entity much before the eighth century B.C. They could not, therefore, vie with the Egyptians in antiquity of race. Nevertheless, the Scythians were a vital political force in their day, and although their history at present occupies only a few lines in some of our more comprehensive reference books, they continue to remain magnificently alive for us as the source of some of our favourite legends. Thus Odysseus' Aeaea or Land of the Rising Sun, the world beyond the grave, is situated in Scythia, on the eastern shores of the Black Sea, in what is now either the Kuban or the Taman peninsula. There too Jason and his Argonauts sought the Golden Fleece, and Odysseus met with his later adventures; it was there that Iphigenia ministered to Diana; thence that Magog set out in fury to cause havoc among the Jews.

In addition to these legends, many strange tales of the wellʼ nigh fabulous wealth of the Scythians came to mingle with the more plausible facts assembled by the Greek historians. So confused was the picture which resulted that, until late in the nineteenth century, many scholars tended even to discount much that Herodotus had written concerning them. Then, gradually, the very high intrinsic value of the objects which were regularly appearing from the Scythian barrows of south ern Russia led archæologists to consult these early records anew.

To their surprise, intermingled with the absurd, they found much that has proved of inestimable value in piecing together a picture of Scythian life. Excavations in our own day continue to produce ever new corroborative evidence in support of some of these ancient assertions, and careful readings of the old texts, combined with the results achieved by spadework in the field, have thrown so much new light on the customs of the steppe nomads of the Scythian age that it has become possible to reconstruct their way of life to an altogether unexpected extent, and to assess with some degree of accuracy the importance of their contribution to the art of western Europe during the Dark Ages.

The Scythians proper actually formed the main clan of a large group of nomads, the tribes of which cannot be clearly differentiated through the references made to them by the early writers. By the seventh century B.C. they had established them‑ selves firmly in southern Russia and the Kuban, and analogous tribes, possibly even related clans, though politically entirely distinct and independent, were also centred on the Altai; some may even have penetrated to the Yenissei district. The origins of these Asiatic tribes cannot now be defined with any degree of certainty, but some of them shared and contributed so much to Scythian art that the entire group, at any rate in the artistic and cultural field, deserves to be considered as one, even though the dissimilarities which occur are often sufficiently marked to warrant differentiation. In these pages, therefore, the term Scythian will be reserved for the specifically Scythian tribes which occupied the Kuban, parts of the Crimea and the great river beds of southern Russia and which, at a somewhat later date, also percolated to Romania, Bulgaria, Hungary and Prussia. The term 'kindred Scyths' will be applied to the nomads of the Altai, and especially to those whose graves have been excavated at Pazirik and on neighbouring sites in the same region. Such a definition has the advantage of not running counter to that of the ancients. Thus, although in accordance with the usage of the late nineteenth century, the term Scythian is reserved by a group of authorities in the USSR for the tribes which ruled over the territory stretching from the Carpathians to the Don, Strabo actually distinguished the region of the Dobrudja as 'Lesser Scythia', while he assigned the whole steppe area lying to the north and north-east of the Black Sea to 'Eastern Scythia'.

Throughout the entire area with which we are concerned, the Scythian and 'kindred Scythian' tribes were basically nomadic, but their pastoral way of life depended to some extent on the existence of agricultural communities, and it is not unlikely that, at any rate by the fifth century B.C., a section of each tribe lived in permanent or semi-permanent encampments which served the nomadic portions of the tribe as a base. The nomads in both the European and the Asiatic sectors of the plain appear to have developed a very similar routine and to have followed closely analogous occupations. As a result there is no very marked difference in the tastes and interests, the clothing and equipment of the two groups. At this distance of time it is impossible to decide how much of the resemblance was due to the existence of definite racial links between the groups, how much to the similarity of their environment and way of life. The art of each, though fundamentally alike, is nevertheless distinguishable because of certain local features resulting in part from the geographical position occupied by each section. The Eurasian steppe is of such immense dimensions, stretching as it does from the edge of the Orient right across to central Europe that, inevitably, peoples living on one or other of its peripheries were bound to come into closer touch with their immediate neighbours, even if they happened to be aliens, than with more distant groups, even if these were kinsmen of their own. Thus, in the east, the influence of China was often to the fore in the nomadic culture of the area, in the centre, Persian elements were more in evidence, and, in the west, those of Greece. Yet in spite of these foreign trends, the nomadic culture predominated throughout, tending to express itself more crudely in the Altai and with greater refinement among the Royal Scyths of southern Russia, and the influences were not entirely in the one direction, for the indigenous culture of the steppe in its turn made itself felt, if to a lesser degree, both in the eastern and the western worlds.

The Scythians formed well-organized communities, responding to their chiefs with ready discipline. But they were a turbulent lot, delighting in warfare, predatory raids and the scalping of their enemies. On more than one occasion their prowess in battle caused real concern to the infinitely more powerful kingdoms of Assyria, Media, Parthia and Greece. In the seventh century B.C. the Scythians were feared throughout Asia Minor, but at the same time their wealth and love of finery won them the good will of the great Hellenic merchants established along the shores of the Black Sea, as well as of the Greek artists and craftsmen who had settled in the Bosphoran kingdom, and more especially at Panticapæum. Even at this early date in their history, the Scythians already displayed an extraordinary ability to appreciate and assimilate the best in the art of their day, regardless of its origin, and they were quick to turn to the highly skilled Greek artists working in the Pontic towns which had sprung up on their southern border in the seventh century B.C., for objects of outstanding quality. The Greeks on their part showed no reluctance to work for the rich nomads on whom they had come to depend for many of their basic foods. The purchases were probably paid for by barter, and from the sixth century B.C. onwards we find the Greeks of the region producing objects which were quite obviously made to the order of Scythian notables. Pieces decorated with scenes from nomad life, which could have been of interest only to the tribal chiefs of the hinterland, have been found and these must have been made as special commissions. We can see much the same thing happening in the south-east, at Sakiz, where, according to Ghirshman,[1] a treasure which had belonged to the Scythian king Partatua or to his son Madyes contained splendid examples of Assyrio-Scythian jewellery.

The Scythians indeed played as active a part in commerce as in war and constituted so important an element in the life of their age that Herodotus found it necessary to devote to them an entire book of his great history. To obtain all possible informa-tion, he set out himself on the tedious journey to Olbia, the Greek outpost city which had been founded in 645 B.C. on the joint mouths of the rivers Bug and Dniestr. Olbia depended for its survival on Scythian protection and on trade with the Scythian world; for the former it paid some form of tribute. Herodotus found it an agreeable and prosperous city and put his time there to good purpose, learning a tribal name from one and hearing of a chieftain's idiosyncrasies from another. He entered it all in the Fourth Book of his History, though he was careful to distinguish between the facts which he had ascertained for himself and the statements reported to him by others, that he had been unable to check. Yet notwith-standing his account, the absence of written documents among the Scythians themselves has proved a strong ally of oblivion, for all memory of the Scythians rapidly faded with their passing from the political scene. By the fourth century A.D. they had been completely forgotten by the civilized world of the day, and some fifteen hundred years were to elapse before their art was rediscovered. It was through this art that they were to become reinstated in the minds of men.

The first step towards reinstatement occurred at the turn of the seventeenth century, when organized bands of grave looters set about a wide-scale robbing of the ancient barrows of Siberia. Reports of their depredations reached Peter the Great. Although too preoccupied in the west to be able to sponsor

[1] Ghirshman (13), p. 106. *The number in parentheses refers to the Bibliography.*

DATE	General Historical Events	Cros... ASIATIC SECTION
700		
600		
500		
400	} Huns evict Goths from S. Russia	
300	} Goths control S. Russia	
200		
100		
A.D.		
B.C.	} Sarmatians control S. Russia	
100	} Kingdom of Neapolis	
200		
300	Sarmatians appear on the Don	
	Chinese cavalry adopt variant of	
400	Nomadic style in dress	Two-way contacts establishe with China. Altai comes in
	Kingdom of the Royal Scyths	touch with Ancient East an
500		Greece by way of Persia
600		
700	Kingdom of Sakiz	
800	} Emperor Suan sets Asiatic tribes in	
900	motion	
1000	{ Mounted nomads appear in Asiatic steppes and Hungarian plain	Chu influence makes itself fe in Siberia
1100	Iron worked at Minussinsk	
1200	Barrow burials in use in Siberia	
1700	Indo-Europeans reach the Yenissei	

Fig. 1. Chronological chart

SOUTH RUSSIAN SECTION	WESTERN EUROPE	DATE
	Scytho-Sarmatian style reflected in art of the Migration period in Central Europe and Gaul. It also influences the Viking art of Scandinavia, thus having an effect on the art of medieval Ireland and England	700
		600
		500
		400
l traces of Scythians disappear	Fleeing Goths spread Scytho-Sarmatian style through Central and S. Europe	300
		200
ythian style revivified by new		100
of polychrome decoration		A.D.
		B.C.
		100
ndency towards naturalism pears in art		200
	Scythians establish outposts in the Balkans	300
		400
	Scythian advance-guards reach E. Germany, Hungary and Bulgaria and come into contact with several Hallstatt tribes	500
yal Scyths firmly established in ropean Russia. Greek influence ns ascendancy in art		600
		700
		800
		900
		1000
		1100
		1200
		1700

controlled excavations in his eastern territories, the Tsar gave explicit orders that the bands were to be broken up, the culprits punished and the objects in their possession dispatched to him at St. Petersburg. In due course a magnificent collection of gold belt buckles and plaques reached the capital. Some were adorned with precious stones or enamels and the majority, following the shape of a horizontal 'B', displayed most curious animal forms. Collectors and art lovers in the capital were completely mystified by the style of the buckles. They were placed in the Tsar's personal treasure room, or Schatzkammer as he called it, and many years later they percolated to what is now the Hermitage Museum at Leningrad, where they still constitute a unique collection of outstanding importance.

Plates 1, 2, 3

During the eighteenth century chance finds in Siberia and southern Russia of objects decorated with animal representations of a somewhat similar character helped to maintain a mild interest in this type of art, which gradually grew to be associated with the nomads of the Eurasian steppe. This view was confirmed in 1763, when General Melgunov, while posted on military duties in southern Russia, opened the magnificent barrows which now bear his name. His discoveries created a stir, but even so, the next real advance in Russian archæology did not occur till the turn of the eighteenth century, when scientific journeys first came to be undertaken in Siberia by such pioneers as Clarke, Pallas, Dubois de Montpéreux, Sumarokov and a score of others. All these travellers noted the multiplicity of early burials which, at any rate for the archæologists, enlivened the seemingly limitless Siberian landscape, but none of them was able to embark on excavations in the area. Nevertheless, in 1806 a Museum was founded at Nikolaev; five years later another was opened at Theodosia; in 1825 one was established at Odessa, and in the following year the most important of all was installed at Kerch. These foundations acted as a spur to antiquarians and within a surprisingly short time two Kerch residents, Dubrux and Stempowski, both of them amateurs, but assisted by the two directors of the Kerch museum, Blaremberg and Ashil, and by the local representative of the Ministry of Interior, Kareisha, tog' ether conducted an excavation on a site close to Kerch. Soon after, similar work was put in hand in the Kuban and in various places close to the southern extremities of the great rivers which intersect the European section of the plain. Very soon it became abundantly clear that the mounds contained not only human and horse burials, but also the products of a marvellously rich group of metal-workers, and that these were to be associated with the Scyths. It likewise became evident that these people had evolved an animal art of considerable individuality, one vibrant with life and impregnated with a static dynamism that defined yet defied the laws of nature by portraying both the real and the imaginary creatures which peopled their fanciful and superstitious minds. Numerous bronze and iron objects were found in the burials, also many made of gold. The latter excited special attention, for it soon became apparent that the decorations on these objects were to some extent related to the buckles from Siberia which Peter the Great had saved from destruction a century or more before.

The next important step in Scythian archæology occurred in the 1860's when V. V. Radlov set out to explore Siberia, this time supplementing surface observations of the mounds by excavations. In 1865 his researches brought him to Katanda, a site in the southern Altai so rich in barrows that he decided to open some of the largest. His interest had been aroused by the unusual construction of these mounds. Instead of being topped with earth, as was generally the case in southern Russia, they were covered with a layer of great boulders. Radlov had been at work on the largest of these mounds for but a short time when his men struck a layer of ice. This was especially surprising since they were in a region which is not subjected to perpetual freezing. Without even suspecting the existence of such a phenomenon, Radlov had stumbled upon the first of the frozen barrows which are now known to be peculiar to this particular area of the Altai.

The formation of ice in these barrows is fortuitous and is due to the layer of stones which caps them. The autumn rains penetrate this layer and filter through the earth beneath; during the intense cold of the winter months the moisture freezes and even in summer this ice, which often freezes to a depth of 21 feet, never melts because of the insulation of the stones above. As a result, many of the bodies and objects buried beneath the layer of ice have been preserved as though in a modern deep-freeze.

Radlov was naturally unaware of the state of affairs, and as he was pressed for time by the lateness of the season, he set about melting the ice as rapidly as possible. As the waters which had been congealed for centuries were released, the astonished archæologist was able to behold the dead with some of their clothes well preserved and their household objects lying virtually intact. But almost as soon as the water penetrated the burial chamber some of the more fragile material disintegrated. Though part was lost, Radlov succeeded in saving most of the tomb's contents, and his finds included articles of clothing and pieces of furniture which were to prove of greater interest some eighty years later than at the time of their discovery.

As excavations in Russia multiplied, producing ever more examples of animal art, it became evident that the whole Eurasian steppe had had a life which stretched far back into the past and that, in the Scythian period, all parts of it had been linked by close and regular contacts. The discovery of gold and metal objects of undoubted Scythian workmanship in the Balkans and in western Europe, however, added new and un-foreseen difficulties to the task of tracing and defining these contacts. Later still, the recognition of Scythian elements in Viking, Celtic and Merovingian art invested the study with even greater complexity, but the difficulties served to spur scholars on. Many archæologists of various nationalities set out to piece the available information together in an endeavour to establish the source and spread of this magnificent nomadic art, to trace the routes of its penetration from zone to zone, and to define its links and influences on other schools of art.

Tolstoy and Kondakov, two eminent Russian antiquarians, were among the first to set to work. They began by listing, describing and attempting to date all Scythian objects extant in Russia. Then Rostovtzeff in Russia, Minns and Dalton in England, Reinach in France, Talgren in Finland, and many more notable scholars besides, studied these findings, compared their own conclusions with the statements of the ancients, and especially with those of Herodotus and Hippocrates, and reached agreement as to the basic facts of Scythian history. The romance of the work gained a strong hold on them, and indeed, no one who has had the good fortune to assist at the opening of a Scythian burial can remain impervious to the fascination of the task. To stand in the translucent air of a day in early sum-mer, the eye roving freely over the plain as it stretches endlessly ahead, changeless and unchanged since the time when the first horseman galloped his steed across its measureless expanse, to stand thus whilst the tomb opens to disclose the fleshless bones of just such another wanderer, with those of his horse lying nearby, their bodies bestrewed with gold ornaments and trap-pings of great intricacy, is an unforgettable experience. It leaves the beholder determined in his turn to try to probe the secrets of an art that is at the same time both curiously abstract and yet basically naturalistic and real.

Rostovtzeff and Minns between them found the answer to many puzzling questions and offered valuable suggestions with regard to others, but many more await solution. Certain

Russian and Hungarian scholars have put forward the interesting idea that the Scythians may have been an Altaic people. This theory has not been generally accepted—indeed, it runs counter to the views of most scholars—yet the results of excavations at Pazirik in the Altai to some extent support it. The recent fieldwork carried out there under the directorship of S. I. Rudenko concerns a kindred tribe and not a purely Scythian one. Nevertheless the similarity between much of the Pazirik material and finds originating from the Kuban and southern Russia is so great that there is often every reason for applying conclusions reached at Pazirik to problems relating to the Scyths, more especially since some of the Pazirik mounds have produced evidence that was hitherto lacking in support of certain passages in Herodotus concerning the Scyths. The Pazirik tombs also show links with those which Radlov examined at Katanda over eighty years ago.

Although the results attained by Radlov at Katanda were scarcely noticed during an age which had been enthralled by such outstanding discoveries as the golden treasures of Pergamon, Troy and Mycenæ, and although they remained unremarked by later archæologists, it is possible that Rudenko had them in mind when he set out in 1924 on an anthropological expedition to Siberia. When chance led him to the very region in the Altai that geologists from the USSR assert alone provides the phenomenon of frozen tombs, he was quick to recognize the possibilities of the various sites which he saw. He was at once impressed by the tombs which abound in the vicinity of the bed of the river Ursul and its tributaries. One valley struck him as especially promising. It was the Pazirik valley, which lies on the southern slopes of the Chulishman range in the Altai mountains. Close to the meeting point of the Pazirik valley and the river Ulagan Rudenko found an important burial ground consisting of some forty mounds. They varied in size and shape, some being round, others oval, but all were topped with the boulders which play so decisive a part in the formation of a protective layer of ice above the burial chamber. Five mounds were exceptionally large and nine of the smaller ones closely resembled them both in shape and construction. In 1929 Rudenko and his colleague Griaznov were able to examine the first of the large barrows. Its contents proved well-nigh sensational, yet the work had to be abandoned at the end of the first season. It was resumed in 1947 and continued for two further years.

By then the excavations had brought to light the story of a people who were not only endowed with an astonishingly acute decorative sense and with an unerring skill for expressing it in a wide variety of materials, but who had also attained to a relatively high degree of culture, involving life in elaborate tents, if not huts, the use of wheeled carts, the ability to ride the horse, to produce elaborate textiles and, to judge from the vessels, quite elaborate cooking. Their art and way of life were rediscovered for us partly as a result of the happy chance which covered their tombs with a protective layer of ice, and also because of the skill and ability with which Rudenko and his assistants overcame the difficulties of excavating in the ice. Rudenko was successful in preserving and transporting his finds without damage from the Altai to the Hermitage Museum. Furthermore, his erudition and sound scholarship enabled him to extract the utmost information from every scrap of evidence likely to have a bearing on the people of Pazirik. Though not nearly as valuable intrinsically as the material from the Royal Scythian tombs of southern Russia, nor from the artistic point of view as satisfying as much of the pure Scythian work from European Russia or Hungary, the Pazirik finds nevertheless throw a great deal more light on the past than do any of the others. As a result, Rudenko's researches pave the way towards establishing a fuller understanding of the art, the life and the history of the peoples of the Eurasian steppe.

CHAPTER I

The Background

THE IMMENSE PLAIN which the tribes of the Scythian and kindred nomads occupied during most of the first millennium stretches from Podolia on the western fringe of European Russia to the borders of China. It forms a single geo-graphical unit of natural grassland, but in Asia it is broken by the Pamirs, the Tien Shan and the Altai ranges, whilst the Urals practically sever the Asian section from the European. *Fig. 2*
Yet communications over the whole vast tract have never been halted by purely geographical obstacles, for two passes, those of Dzungaria and Ferghana, form corridors which connect the Asiatic and European portions of the plain. In prehistoric times the grass covered virtually the whole of the central Asian section but certain climatic changes occurred there a little before the dawn of the historic period and as a result, large areas of pasture were transformed into barren, sand-covered deserts unfit for habitation. But these sandy stretches remained open to travel, their transformation failing to impede the movements of the steppe dwellers or to curb the inter-tribal contacts which had been established. Thus relationships between tribes persisted on traditional lines from the earliest until quite recent times.

In antiquity the boundaries of the region with which we are concerned were defined by geographical features rather than by political demarcation lines. Moving from east to west, they consisted of the Nan Shan and Tien Shan ranges, and the Oxus river; the Iranian plateau which succeeded them was perhaps more of a political frontier, but it was followed again by natural boundaries, formed in turn by the Caucasian mountains, the Black Sea, the Carpathians and the river Danube. Along the steppe's northern fringe uninviting, dangerous lands covered with sinister marshes, vast forests and

C

wild tundra were inhabited by fierce Finno-Ugrian tribesmen, but the natural perils of the countryside were in themselves sufficient to serve as powerful deterrents to Scythian penetration.

Then as now, the Asiatic section of the steppe was subjected to intense cold during the winter months and to torrid heat in the summer, and in consequence the vegetation of that region has always been less luxuriant and less well suited to primitive methods of agriculture than that of southern Russia. Though cedars flourished on many Asiatic hillsides, pines, larch and birch were common to both areas. Annuals and biennials were, however, practically unknown to the Asiatic section, whereas, in southern Russia, the steppe was carpeted with flowers throughout the spring. In Asia much of the vegetation con-sisted of plants of the Gramineæ family, such as *Festucata sulcata, Avena desertorum* and *Trisetum flavescens. Potentillas fruticosa* and *subacaulis* also grew there. Equally common were *Antennaria dioica, Leontopodium sibiricum, Artemisia sacrorum* and *Senecio pratensis* of the Compositæ group. Sanfoin, wild thyme, *Aconitum barbatum, Pulsatilla patens* and Anemones of various varieties flourished, and *Schizonepeta multifida* and *Phlomis tuberosa* covered great patches of ground. In the spring, *Iris ruthenica* and *Dianthus seguieri* often gladdened the eye. In south-ern Russia the land was more thickly afforested and oaks, limes, ashes and acacias spread their shade over much of the plain, fruit trees afforded a welcome harvest, and splendid grass served to fatten the herds. Edible roots and bulbs furnished mankind with food, coriander was obtainable for the making of infusions and hemp provided a narcotic, potent both as a medicament and as a stimulant capable of inducing sensations amounting to ecstasy.

The entire region was tremendously rich in animal life. In Asia elks, bears, wolves, leopards, bison and wild horses roamed in the steppe. In Europe wild boars, asses, goats, otters and beavers were common. Susliks, tiny creatures of the jerboa family, and hares, minks and ermine scudded in the under-growth; adders and snakes lurked in the grass, and bees, which were valued for their honey, zoomed above. Eagles, pheasants, francolins and many birds besides filled the sky. All these animals and birds, together with many others, appear in Scythian art, often powerfully stylized, though still clearly recognizable with all their essential features and characteristics triumphantly preserved, or else altered into mythical creatures so strange that the original beast is often completely transformed.

The European section of the steppe was in general more lush, clement and fertile than the Aisatic. It was traversed by great rivers—the Volga, the Don with its tributary the Donetz, the Dniepr, the Bug and finally the Dniestr—all of which provided immense hauls of fish and valuable salt deposits. Their waters fertilized the valleys, but did not impede movement unduly. The nomads were thus able to roam at will across the entire region, either pasturing their cattle or pursuing the game in which the steppe abounded, without having to contend with any serious geographical obstacles and without encountering any startling changes in climate or vegetation. For just as the character of the Asiatic sector had undergone modification in early prehistoric times owing to changes of climate, so too has the temperature of the European portion altered since the classical age. Southern Russia has thus tended to become warmer and drier than it was when the Greeks of the Bosphoran kingdom were in the habit of complaining of the cold and wet on the northern shores of the Black Sea. In their day the Caspian was undoubtedly very much larger than in Christian times. It is very probable that it used to jut out south of Krasnovodsk into the large gulf which Ellsworth Hunting-ton[1] identifies with the Scythian Gulf referred to by Diodorus of Sicily in about the year 60 B.C. In those days the Oxus must have flowed into this gulf, for the trade route from the west to the east followed its river bed. When the Caspian contracted, the river must have altered its course, turning towards the Sea of Aral. Parts of the reduced Caspian were probably then used for habitation, but as the lands dried out, food supplies must have decreased until the herds had to be thinned out and the nomad population was forced to contract.

Good building stone was scarce in the western sector, though one or two rich outcrops were worked in classical times in the Crimea and limestone was also quarried at Kerch. From about the eighth century B.C. small supplies of iron were obtained from the region of the central Dniepr, but large amounts were procured from the Caucasus, where it was so plentiful that the Greeks thought that it had been invented there. Copper was also mined in immense amounts in Transcaucasia and gave rise among the Greeks to their tales about the Argonauts, but gold came partly from the north-east of the Urals, and mainly from the very rich Altaian mines. In view of the distance involved, it is a little surprising that the Scythians in the western region of the steppe seem to have had unlimited supplies of gold at their disposal. Their stocks could only have come from their fellow tribesmen to the east, and indeed nothing could have been easier than the establishment of a gold trade between the two zones; it must in fact have existed from an early date. There is nothing to show how the Scythians paid for this gold. The Royal Scyths may have done so with the metal coinage they evolved from Greek prototypes, but the kindred tribes may have used plain, as opposed to trefoil arrow-heads as currency. The problem remains unsolved.

It is curious too that although amber was found in small quantities in the vicinity of Kiev, it was imported from the Adriatic and was most widely used in the Kuban. Shells were very scarce in all areas, yet some graves contained cowrie shells that must have come from the Indian Ocean.

In neolithic times, whilst the inhabitants of western Asia were still hunters, their contemporaries on the Amu Darya were fishermen who had come in contact with the cultivators of Merv and had learnt to produce for themselves some red and black pottery and also perhaps some woven stuffs. In Europe at much the same time, the inhabitants of wood and wattle houses in the Ukraine were decorating their pots with geometric patterns, and a very little later Tripolje pottery displayed figures of bulls, goats, dogs, stags and men. In Siberia succeeding generations painted their pottery with red or white bands resembling to some extent that of Susa or Sialk, they kept large domestic animals, and they placed their dead with legs bent, in rectangular graves covered with a stone slab. According to Kiselev[2], it was between the years 3000 and 1700 B.C. that the first agriculturalists to work the soil of Siberia, coming from the west, settled on the more fertile lands. Paradoxically, it is at very much the same date that pastoral nomads first appeared in the Ukraine. The latter were fair-haired men of the long-headed type, quite probably Thracians; they carried battle-axes of European shape, they had domesticated the horse and, before burial, they daubed their dead with an ochre paint which stained even their bones a reddish colour. This was a period of immense movements of peoples, tribes from the west heading eastward and those in the east making for the west. There must have been some widespread cause for these migrations; possibly one of the great droughts which used periodically to affect most of eastern Europe and western Asia. This opening phase in the migratory movement was to culminate a thousand years later with the appearance in southern Europe of two distinct cultures, the Scythian in southern Russia and the Etruscan in Italy, for even though they were completely divorced and separate civilizations, they were not wholly alien.

In so far as the Scythians were concerned, the initial point in their history can perhaps be assigned to about 1700 B.C., when the first Indo-European tribes reached the Yenissei. These migrants may have broken away from the Indo-European group which had penetrated to Greece and Asia Minor some three centuries earlier. From the Yenissei they advanced west of the Altai to the Caucasus, where Kiselev[3] believes that they evolved a mixed economy for themselves, some of the tribe settling as agriculturists in the fertile valleys, while the rest roamed the plain as pastoral nomads and hunters. The settlers had by then mastered the art of casting and forging copper, and some of their foundries have been discovered sunk in the earth, with the moulds they used for making their sickles lying close at hand. They produced a brownish pottery on which they scratched geometric designs, and used bronze celts for cutting down trees. At first they buried their dead in flattish graves marked with a circle of boulders, but towards 1200 B.C., they began to construct great barrows. Kiselev[4] believes that the difference in size of the barrows erected side by side on a single burial ground depended on the clan's wealth, but since the dissimilar barrows contain graves which appear to belong to people of a common race or clan it is tempting to ascribe the difference in scale to the emergence of a class society, with families of substance and power expecting to be treated with special consideration in death as in life.

At much the same date tribes in north-eastern Siberia began to use iron, and at Minussinsk, situated in the Yenissei basin, a new Mongoloid race appeared, equipped with inward curving knives resembling those which are associated with the Chu dynasty of China. The presence of this shape marks the penetration of Chinese influence to a region which had until then been mainly affected by trends from western Asia or eastern Europe. This group of people either cremated their dead, burying their ashes beneath a stone slab, or sometimes they laid the body there instead, arranging it in a crouching position. No horse skeletons are found in association with them, and it must therefore be assumed that, like the Chinese themselves, the people who were among the first to introduce orientalism to the west had not as yet learnt to ride the horse. Mounted nomads, amongst them Scythian and Masemir tribesmen from the Altai were, however, prominent at this time in other sections of the Asiatic steppe. The more important individuals of these groups had their riding horses buried beside them. In Europe, though some horsemen, possibly men of Thracian stock, had appeared in Hungary towards 1000 B.C., unmounted Cim-merians still continued to control southern Russia.

Of the various tribes of horsemen who are associated with central Asia and eastern Europe, the Scythians were eventually to prove the most important both in their own day and also in the Dark Ages, when their influence made itself felt in the art of northern and western Europe. Yet at this distance of time it is impossible to determine the exact racial group to which the Scythians belonged. The problem has given rise to much con-troversy, some authorities asserting that they were Huns, others that they were Turks or Mongols. In the main, however, most scholars agree that they were people of the Indo-European group, possibly of Iranian stock or, as Géza Nagy[5] and some others suggest, Ugro-Altaians. The only indubitable fact which emerges is that the tribes of the entire plain all spoke the same language, in much the same way that many present-day nomads throughout Asia all speak the Turki dialect of Turk-ish. The language spoken by the nomads was basically an Iranian tongue, but it may have been more closely allied to Avestic than to ancient Persian.[6]

There is very little anthropological material which can help to throw light on the problem, but what is available seems to support the Indo-European attribution, and this does not in its turn exclude an Altaian designation. An examination of the male skulls and mummified heads found at Pazirik confirms this view, notwithstanding that the chieftain buried in Mound 2 and a woman from one of the other burials were both Mon-goloid in type, as was also an old man buried in an interesting,

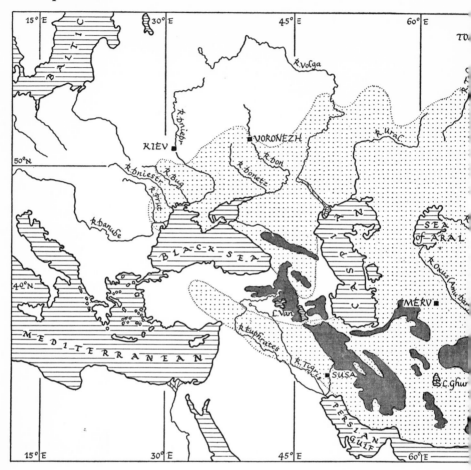

Fig. 2. Physical m

somewhat similar grave at Shibe in the Altai, excavated by Griaznov in 1927.[7] Indeed, there is nothing surprising in the occasional presence of people of Mongol blood among the tribes inhabiting the eastern section of the Asiatic steppe, for there was probably intermarriage between them and the locals,

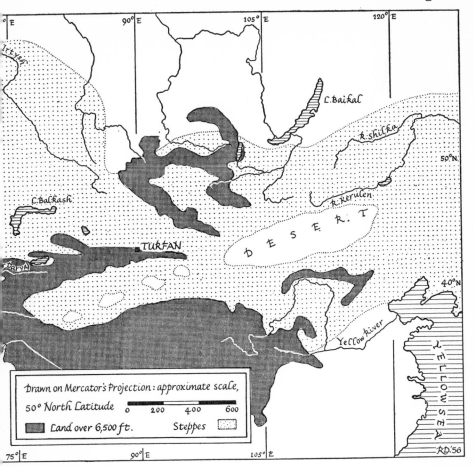

Scythian influence.

just as the Royal Scyths at times intermarried with Greeks or Thracians from neighbouring regions in the west. The union of weak and powerful tribes by marriage was often the only way of ensuring the security of the smaller clan. Thus King Ariapeithes of southern Russia married a Greek woman from

41

Istrus, as well as a Scythian and also the daughter of the Thracian chief Teres.

The ancient Greeks applied the names Scyth, Saka or Caha indiscriminately to all the nomads of the Eurasian steppe, with/ out distinguishing between those inhabiting lands within reach of China and those living close to the Carpathians. As late as the second century A.D. Ptolemy called Sineria in central Asia, Scythia. Herodotus, whom time has proved correct in much that he wrote about the Scythians, thought that they had all come from Asia and that, at an unspecified date, the Asiatic Scythians had split from those living on the Euxine. Present/ day scholars in the USSR use the term Scythian in its narrow/ est sense, applying it only to the comparatively small number of tribes who lived on the shores of the Sea of Azov, the Black Sea, the Kuban and the Dniepr. But since all the mounted nomads of the Scythian age spoke the same Iranian tongue, whether they came from the Dniestr or the banks of the Oxus, there seems reason to think that at any rate the majority were linked by some sort of racial tie. A definite affinity is indeed suggested by the nature of their art, which shows well/nigh identical features over so wide an area. The presence of certain seemingly Siberian elements in the west lends support to the view held by some scholars that the Scythians were a west/Siberian, or as Minns and Géza Nagy hint, a specifically Altaic people. Final confirmation of this belief will, however, depend on whether future excavations in the Altai produce material of the Scythian type older in date than anything found in the Kuban and southern Russia. So far, this has not been the case.

There is thus as much divergence of opinion regarding the original area of habitation of the Scythians as there is over their racial origin. Yet if an Altaic or west/Siberian attribution proves acceptable with regard to the ethnic problem, then the tribes' subsequent migrations from that area become more readily understandable. This view has, moreover, the additional advantage of not running counter to the statements which occur in ancient Persian documents. According to these sources, many of which are contemporary with the events they describe, the Scythians made a sudden appearance, advancing from the north-west across the Caucasus. This belief was shared by Greek, Jewish and Armenian writers, and it represents the considered opinion of the ancient world.

It likewise tallies with the march of certain well authenticated events in Chinese history as related in the annals of the Chu dynasty. These concern the wild Hiung-nu tribesmen, the forerunners, as it is thought, of those very Huns who were later to devastate so much of Europe, and who, already at this early date, were harassing the peaceful agriculturalists of China's western frontier lands. By the ninth century B.C. they were causing such extensive damage that the emperor Suan (827-781 B.C.) felt obliged to take military action against them. His punitive expedition succeeded in pushing the Hiung-nu well to the west of China's borders. A purely defensive measure, it was destined to have unexpectedly widespread repercussions in areas many hundreds of miles to the west of the battlefield, for the retreating Hiung-nu inevitably dislodged their western neighbours from their traditional camping grounds. These in their turn cannoned into the next tribe, which duly lashed out against the tribe living on its western flank, so that the entire steppe was soon in motion, each tribe attacking its western neighbour in an effort to secure new pastures. Yet it is signifi- cant that the unrest corresponds to the severe drought assigned by Ellsworth Huntington to about the year 800 B.C.[8] and this may well have served as a contributory factor in the westward migratory movement.

At any rate the Massagatæ, who lived to the north of the Oxus, eventually became involved in the struggle for pastoral lands, and they in their turn assaulted the Scythians, who attacked the eastern Cimmerians. In the battle which ensued between the latter combatants, the Scythians, who were mounted on horses, proved superior to the Cimmerians, who fought on foot. The Cimmerians found themselves pushed back towards the Dariel pass and were forced to retreat through it. This led them to the kingdom of Van and Urartu, a rival and enemy of Assyria. The Scythians on their part continued to press forward, one detachment crossing either the Jaxartes or the Volga, passing thence into southern Russia, where it found and conquered the main body of Cimmerians, whilst another group, turning aside from the Dariel Pass, headed for the Derbend Defile, emerging from it on the shores of Lake Urmia. Assyrian documents place their appearance there in the time of King Sargon (722/705 B.C.), a date which closely corresponds with that of the establishment of the first group of Scythians in southern Russia. This date can therefore be considered as marking the final stage in the westerly migration of Asiatic tribes which had been set in motion by the emperor Suan's punitive measures against the Hiung-nu. In Armenia, the ruined walls of some ancient forts still hold the Scythians' trefoil arrow-heads embedded in their mortar as testimony of the bitter fighting.

Further Scythian advances into Asia must be regarded as purely military ventures, for the Scythians could have settled on lake Urmia had they wished to do so. However, exhilarated by their success, they continued steadily to press the Cimmerians back towards Asia and another thirty years brought the combatants to the borders of Assyria. The Scythians then allied themselves with King Esarhadon in his fight against the Medes, but, aided by some renegade Cimmerians, they themselves concentrated against their original enemy, pushing the main body of Cimmerians back across Asia Minor till, by 635 B.C., they had broken their opponent. The fleeing Cimmerians retreated over Phrygian territory belonging to King Midas. This they utterly destroyed, then they overran Lydia and sacked the Greek coastal cities. After that they disappear from sight.

Meanwhile, in the area roughly corresponding to present-day Azerbaidzhan, the kingdom of Urartu had crumbled. The Scythians under their king Partatua and his son Madyes, firmly established themselves in northern Persia, occupying Urartu itself, where they set up their capital at Sakiz, and controlling other territory as far west as the Halys. Their might seemed very great at that time, and in 626 B.C. their aid enabled the Assyrians to break the Median siege of Nineveh. Intoxicated by their success, the Scythians pressed on, sweeping across Syria and Judæa till they reached Philistæa in Egypt (611 B.C.), where any further advance was bought off by King Psamatek. In the meantime, however, the Medes had allied themselves with the Babylonians. Their joint armies advanced against the Assyrians and this time their united forces succeeded in destroying this once mighty empire. The Medes then promptly assumed power, making it their first task to evict the Scythians from their land, and not resting till they had pushed the nomads steadily back across Asia to the point from which they had started their invasion of Persia. As the price of their clemency, they wisely insisted that some of the tribal horsemen should be left to settle in the province of Luristan, there to train and establish cavalry units for the Median army.

The Scythians had ruled a large portion of western Asia for twenty-eight years. They were now back in Urartu. It was perhaps at this date that some turned eastward again, to occupy the tract of steppe lying between the Caspian and the Sea of Aral, blending there with their Dahai kinsmen to form the ethnic group from which the Parthians were to spring some three hundred years later. Others may have pushed on as far as India, thus accounting for the Scythian admixture in the Scytho-Dravidians, whilst others remained in Armenia. The majority, however, made for the western steppe, where they found their kinsmen prosperously and firmly established on the fertile lands of southern Russia.

In the following century it fell to the western Scyths to be-come involved in a major war. Their attacker was no less a general than the mighty Darius. He had determined to conquer and utterly destroy Greece, and as a first step he set out to cut her vital supplies, particularly her timber imports from the Balkans and her consignments of grain from Scythia. With this end in view, in either the year 516 or 513 B.C., he launched a campaign in Europe, crossing the Bosphorus over a bridge which had been specially built for him by the ingenious Greek engineer, Mandrocles of Samos. The next stage carried him across Thrace to the Danube. This too he crossed by means of a bridge of boats thrown across the river a little below the present-day Galatz. Leaving a detachment of Ionians with instructions to guard it for sixty days pending his return, failing which they were to retire across it, destroying it behind them, he proceeded to seek out the Scythians. But at the first alert the nomads realized that they could not stand up unaided against Darius in open battle. They appealed to neighbouring tribes for help, attempting to persuade them into an alliance by arguing that safety lay in numbers, for whereas Darius could destroy them all singly, he would find it difficult to conquer them if they united. But the northerners were not to be persuaded, pre-ferring to hope for a reprieve rather than to court battle against so skilled a general. Obliged therefore to rely on their own resources, the Scythians decided to seek safety in a scorched earth policy. According to custom, they divided their army into three groups, each commanded respectively by one of the three Royal Scyths, Idanthyrsus, Scopasis and Taxacis. They agreed that whichever of the three was pursued by Darius would retreat into the interior, breaking up the wells and denuding the land of food and fodder.

Darius took the offensive by crossing the Don and marching towards the Volga. The Scyths steadily retreated before him. The sixty days which the Persian had set his Ionian guards as a time limit for defending the bridge across the Danube were fast slipping away, his men were wearying of the profitless chase, his animals were running short of fodder, yet the Scyths continued to retreat ever farther eastward. Their unwillingness to give battle exasperated Darius. He determined to force the issue and he challenged Idanthyrsus in the following words: 'Thou strange man,' shouted his messenger, 'why dost thou keep on flying before me, when there are two things thou mightest do so easily? If thou deemest thyself able to resist my arms, cease thy wanderings and come, let us engage in battle. Or if thou art conscious that my strength is greater than thine—even so thou shouldest cease to run away—thou hast but to bring thy lord earth and water, and to come at once to a conference.' But the Scythian king proudly replied: 'This is my way, Persian. I never fear men or fly from them. I have not done so in the past, nor do I fly from thee. There is nothing new or strange in what I do; I only follow my common mode of life in peaceful years. Now I will tell thee why I do not at once join battle with thee. We Scythians have neither towns nor cultivated lands, which might induce us, through fear of their being taken or ravaged, to be in any hurry to fight you. If, however, you must needs come to blows with us speedily, look you now, there are our fathers' tombs—seek them out and attempt to meddle with them—then ye shall see whether or no we will fight with you. Till ye do this, be sure we shall not join battle unless it pleases us. This is my answer to the challenge to fight.'9

Disheartened, realizing that further pursuit was useless, Darius decided to withdraw. The Scythians harassed his retreating men, but the Persian succeeded in getting his troops back to the bridge and across the Danube to safety. The expedition was at an end. Darius had escaped disaster, but he never again ventured into northern Europe.

The infuriated Scythians were left longing for revenge. Aristagorus had now become their leader. Assembling his forces he advanced on Abydos and appealed to King Cleo-menes I of Sparta to march against the Persians from Ephesus whilst he advanced against them from Phasis, but Darius succeeded in burning Abydos and Cleomenes refused to become involved in the fighting. Aristagorus had perforce to abandon his plan. After plundering Thrace in 495 B.C., he advanced instead on Chersonesus, put its tyrant Miltiades to flight, and then withdrew to his lands, where his men resumed their peaceful occupations and petty, inter-tribal skirmishes.

In the following century the Royal Scyths became conscious of a new tribe, the Sarmatian, which had appeared on the eastern fringe of their territory and had begun to encroach upon their lands. The Sarmatians were a tribe of very similar origin to the Scythians. Both shared the same language and an almost identical way of life, but Sarmatian maidens rode, hunted and fought with their men-folk, whereas Scythian women lived a life of complete retirement and seclusion, taking no part in the activities of the men. Indeed, no Sarmatian girl could wed until she had killed a foe in battle, and it was perhaps because of this that the Scythians spoke of these girls as 'the lords of men'. Yet once they had killed their man, the women were given in marriage and had thenceforth entirely to devote them-selves to domestic occupations.

Although the Greeks associated their stories of the Amazons with the Scythians, it is far more probable that they in fact referred to the Sarmatians. In this connection the chance discovery in 1928 by a group of agricultural workers of a grave at Zemo-Avchala, eight miles or so from Tiflis, belonging to a woman-warrior is of considerable interest. The woman had been buried in a crouching position and her weapons were put close beside her. No comparable graves of a Scythian character have as yet been found in Russia, and Nikoradze,[10] who published the burial, is almost certainly correct in dating it to the third century B.C. Although he did not attribute it to any particular tribe, it is more than probable that this unusual tomb was that of a Sarmatian Amazon. She may well have died in the struggle against the Scythians.

By 346 B.C., the aggressiveness of the Sarmatians had carried them across the Don, and it may have been the wish to find safer lands which induced the Scythian king Ateas to lead his men across the Danube and annex those areas of the Dobrudja that classical writers came to refer to as 'Lesser Scythia'. By the year 339 B.C. the Scythians had advanced to a point a little to the west of modern Balchik, thereby drawing upon themselves the irritation of Philip II of Macedon. Fearing their further infiltration, Philip met them in battle at a point close to the Danube and succeeded in killing Aertes, who was over ninety years old at the time. The Scythians had to agree to peace terms, but they cannot fully have adhered to them, for within three years Alexander the Great in his turn felt forced to send a punitive expedition against them. Setting out himself for the main theatre of war in Asia, he dispatched his Thracian governor, Zepyrion, to deal with the Scythians, but the unfortunate man proved unequal to the task. His troops were routed, he himself was killed in the battle and the Scythians established tribute-paying outposts in the Balkans before returning to their own kingdom in southern Russia. They would have preferred to have stayed on to continue the fight against the Macedonians, and had even appealed to Olbia for help in doing so, but this was refused them. Realizing their weakness, they decided to let the fighting peter out.

Nevertheless, the Scythians soon rallied again. Their king Scylurus established his capital at Neapolis in about 110 B.C. and, like the autonomous rulers of Lesser Scythia of much the same date,[11] he struck his own coins at Olbia. Despite the serious menace which the Sarmatians now presented, he could not resist attacking Chersonesus, even though it was the capital of Mithridates Eupator of the Pontus. Mithridates, who was to remain master of the whole of Asia Minor until the year 95 B.C., had little difficulty in repulsing the Scythians, but before any truly decisive results had been reached in the fighting he found that he had become so deeply involved in his simultaneous contest against Rome that he sought a Scythian alliance. To propitiate Scylurus he dispatched two of his daughters to him as brides, but before the unfortunate girls were able to reach their destination, they were captured by the Romans, and the help which the Scythians afterwards gave to Mithridates was but intermittent and slight. Indeed, they were now in no position to do much more, for the Sarmatians, like the Scythians themselves some seven hundred years earlier, were relentlessly pushing westward across the Eurasian steppe. Also like the Scythians before them, the Sarmatian warriors were to achieve complete success in their advance by reason of their new equipment, for whereas the Scythians had conquered because of the advantages which they derived from their ability to ride the horse, the Sarmatians did so by inventing the metal stirrup, which in its turn facilitated the establishment of heavy cavalry units in the army. The Scythians were beaten by the more modern force. Pockets of them lingered on here and there until the second century A.D., when the majority were wiped out by the Goths, the next wave of people to advance across southern Europe. Other groups of Scythians were no doubt so completely assimilated by the local inhabitants that they left behind them only a few traces of the strange blend of turbulence and splendour which had characterized their lives.

In their heyday the Scythians were a prosperous people, obtaining much of their wealth from trade, more especially from trade with Greece, for even in those far distant days

Hellas was already unable to feed her mainland population without importing basic necessities from far afield. Scythia served as one of Greece's granaries, and in southern Russia the corn grown by the settlers was transmitted by the nomadic overlords to the Greek colonists of the Pontus, who in their turn acted as middlemen in selling it to Greece. The Scythians in the Kuban, on the other hand, traded direct with the masters of vessels coming to their ports from Ionia. In addition, the Scyths as a whole supplied the Pontic Greeks with valuable consignments of salt, sturgeon and tunny-fish, with honey, meat and milk, hides and furs, and not least important, with slaves. The latter, though described by the Greeks as 'Scythians', were probably conquered enemies or local agriculturalists rather than nomad freemen. In return for this merchandise the Scythians received Greek jewellery, metalwork and pottery of the finest quality.

In Europe each of the main groups of Scythians seems to have had a special period of magnificence. The Kuban group was one of the first to be able to indulge its love of opulence and pomp to the full. Its burials, the finest of which are to be dated between the early seventh and late sixth century B.C., contain magnificent objects in gold, many of them examples of the finest workmanship, and in this region the horses killed at the death of a single chief often ran into hundreds. Although the Scythians of this area followed a patriarchal rule, electing their chief as was doubtless done at Pazirik, many of the tombs are so rich that it is probable that a fair number of the more prosperous families were almost as wealthy as their chieftains.

In southern Russia the political structure was slightly different. There, the Scythians considered themselves autochthonous, believing that they were descended from patriarch Targitaus, the son of the God of Heaven and the half-woman, half-serpent daughter of the river Dniepr. According to the Scythian account, recorded by Herodotus, a golden plough, a yoke, a battle-axe and a cup—all four of which denoted sovereignty over husbandmen and warriors alike—fell from heaven. The sons of Targitaus advanced to pick up these objects, but as the two eldest approached, flames sprang up driving them back. When the youngest son came forward the flames died down, so he took the emblems and became king of the royal tribe of Phalatæ and the nation of Scolot. This son, Colaxis by name, later divided his kingdom between his own three sons, and the system of dividing the kingdom's fighting forces into three groups persisted for many centuries, just as the core of the kingdom continued to centre round the region stretching from the lower Dniepr to the river Tokmak, a tributary of the Molochnaya.

The legend is, of course, little more than a variant of the Iranian version of the halo of majesty which could fall only to a pious king. The Scythians also believed that Targitaus had lived a thousand years prior to 513 B.C., that is to say many centuries before the Scythians themselves reached the Dniepr. Owing to the legend, they concentrated the royal tombs within the terri-tory they associated with Targitaus and continued tacitly to recognize the hereditary succession of their leaders, for in their case the ruler was more of a king than a chieftain. This naturally led to the growth of an aristocracy within the area, and it also resulted in an increase in the personal wealth of the royal and princely families. This wealth is observable in the graves of the area, for the royal tombs are the richest of all the Scythian burials, containing more gold and other precious materials than have been found anywhere else in the Eurasian steppe.

The Royal Scyths were relatively few in number, but they were such efficient rulers and such fearless fighters that they had no difficulty in governing a large territory and controlling with ease a population consisting of their own husbandmen and the indigenous agriculturalists whom they had found established in the region, and who greatly outnumbered them. Regardless of the disparity in numbers, by the sixth century B.C., and possibly even as much as a hundred years earlier, the Royal Scyths were already firmly established in the area bounded by the Don and the Dniepr, and virtually controlled the steppe as far west as the Bug and the productive lands in the neighbour-hood of Poltava. In these lands they ruled as despots. A man over whom the sovereign had pronounced the death penalty died together with all his male relatives, it being the law that none should survive who might institute a blood feud. Yet if a king displeased his bodyguard, they likewise did not hesitate to put him to death. King Scyles, himself the son of a Greek woman, thus paid for his philhellene sympathies with his life, for his admiration for Greek culture led him to participate in the Dionysian celebrations being held in one of the Pontic cities of the region. His bodyguard were bitterly angered by an act which they regarded as a defection. They broke into the town and murdered the unfortunate king as he left the temple.

Yet many Scythian aristocrats persisted in finding delight in Greek culture and in admiring the finest Greek works of art. Some amongst them were fascinated by Greek thought and religion, others were charmed by the beauty of Greek urban architecture, members of the royal house being often the ones who were most attracted by the Greek way of living. King Scyles was among the first of the nomads to acquire a house. He chose it in Olbia and adorned its façade with spectacular figures of the sphinxes and griffins which the Scythians held in particular affection. The rank and file, however, remained obstinately conservative and nationalist, and although the Royal Scyths were the recognized protectors of many of the Pontic cities, yet, whether they wished it or not, the kings continued to live in camps in the traditional way, residing there surrounded by their princes and cavalrymen, their cattle and huntsmen.

The Scythian aristocracy was accepted as readily by the local, indigenous settlers of the area as by the pastoral and agricultural

Scythians. Officials and minor chiefs lived in much the same manner as the king and chieftains, though on a smaller scale. For administrative purposes Royal Scythia or Scythia proper was divided into four districts, each of which was controlled by a governor holding his appointment from the king. Amongst other duties, it fell to the governors to collect the prescribed tributes from the agriculturalists of their district as well as from certain Pontic cities which, like Olbia, were liable for tribute. They had too to attend a yearly gathering of the warriors, when those who had killed their first enemy drank the victim's blood in the presence of the governor and a crowd of envious and admiring spectators. The Scythians actually believed that only in this way could they incorporate the dead enemy's valour with their own. The governors were provided with troops who were paid in kind, in contrast to the bodyguard of a chieftain. The latter were freemen chosen from among the tribesmen, and though they were not paid soldiers, they were entitled to a share of the day's loot, but after battle each warrior had to show his chief the severed head of an enemy for only then was he entitled to his share. In time of war, the forces drawn from the three sections into which the country was then divided were split into companies, each of which had its own commander. Once a year the companies assembled with their officers to feast with their king. Any man who had either killed an enemy in the sight of his king or who had won a lawsuit in the king's hearing was entitled to preserve the skull of his dead foe. According to Herodotus, the Scythians often scalped their enemies, sometimes making a napkin of the skin and invariably turning the skulls into mugs, mounting them in gold or some other precious material and wearing them suspended from their belts. They used them for drinking blood brotherhood vows[12] or for sealing an oath, pledging themselves in a mixture of wine and blood in which they had first dipped the tips of their swords.

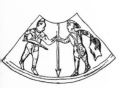

Fig. 3.
A cap from the Kurdzhip barrows, Kuban, showing two Scythian warriors. One holds the severed head of an enemy. IV—III c. B.C. Length, about 7½ in.

Herodotus refers to a group of rebel Scyths who had broken away from the main clan and migrated to the north-west of Lake Balkash, settling in an area which he called Sacæ. It seems probable that pockets of other equally independently-minded Scyths existed elsewhere in the steppe, and it may even have been dissenters similar to these who penetrated to Prussia, thus accounting for burials of what appear to be single warriors such as that of Vettersfeld. Although the majority of the Scythian settlements in the Balkans should perhaps be regarded as outposts which had been intentionally established by the Royal Scyths, rather than as single penetrations similar to that of Vettersfeld, some of the earlier Scythian burial grounds lying on Hungarian soil seem, on the other hand, to be associated with adventurous groups restlessly pushing ever farther towards the west. The position is somewhat different with regard to the later burials which survive in Romania and Bulgaria, for these may have belonged to small groups of Scythians who had abandoned their south Russian pastures in an effort to escape from the Sarmatians relentlessly advancing from the east. All these far-flung groups adhered to the customs and beliefs of their forebears and preserved much of the original purity of their very personal artistic traditions.

Sources

Numbers in parentheses refer to the Bibliography on p. 201.

1 Ellsworth Huntington (9), p. 335.

2 Kiselev (81), pp. 48, 61, 94.

3 *Ibid.*, p. 104.

4 *Ibid.*, p. 228.

5 Géza Nagy (100).

6 Vasmer (51).

7 Kiselev (81), p. 182.

8 Ellsworth Huntington (9), p. ix.

9 Herodotus (15), Book IV.

10 Nikoradze (86).

11 Tarassuk (97), pp. 22–30.

12 For a contemporary pictorial representation of two Scyths drinking brotherhood vows from a single cup see Minns (18), fig. 98, p. 203.

CHAPTER II

The People

A T FIRST GLANCE a tribesman's life is very apt to charm an onlooker by its apparent freedom from care and responsibility. This is, however, no more than a superficial impression, resulting largely from the nomad's happy-go-lucky disposition, which is itself the fortunate result of his strictly limited requirements. On reflection, it very soon becomes apparent that nomads have to follow a discipline no less rigorous than that which regulates the lives of sedentary communities, even though it is a discipline of its own.

A nomad's prosperity, if not his very survival, hinges on his ability to meet his needs, and the well-being of the tribe as a whole, and in consequence its efficiency and vitality, rests upon the ease with which they are satisfied. This in turn depends to a very great extent upon the organizing ability and foresight of the tribal chieftain, and also on the readiness with which individual tribesmen respond to his orders. A successful leader is a man of considerable acumen, one able to handle men and plan ahead, one who is at the same time an opportunist and deft at coming to a quick decision. A community which spends its life in the open, virtually unprotected from the fiercest vicissitudes of the weather and ever at the mercy of the many hazards that lurk in wild, uninhabited country has but itself and its chief to rely on, and anyone who has watched such a group of people on the move, be it the Bedouins of the Arab world, the Turki tribes of central Asia or the nomads who roamed pre-revolutionary Russia, has quickly come to realize that there is no room for the improvident and irresponsible in such conditions. Even a picnic requires forethought if it is to prove a success. A migration demands an infinitely greater effort from all concerned in it, for adaptability and co-ordination are both equally necessary if the daily move is to get under way efficiently and swiftly, ensuring the smooth and even tenure of a form of life which follows a pattern as complex as that of any settled society.

Most nomads are cattle breeders and rely on their herds for their food and clothing. Good pasture land is thus their first need, the very prerequisite of their lives, and the tribe as a whole is therefore always ready to contest its hold on such land and if necessary to defend it. In normal times pastures are not seized haphazardly in a seasonal scramble, nor obtained in an annual free fight, but by tradition they are associated with particular tribes, the boundaries of the territories being as clearly estab-lished and their ownership as precisely known as are those of arable fields amongst agricultural communities. In consequence a tribe often spends years in the same district, moving with the seasons from the same winter pastures to the same summer grasslands as their fathers have done for generations previously. Then an unforeseen change, some climatic disaster, such as soil erosion or desiccation, or an act of aggression by a neighbour, deprives the tribe of its customary territory. In the ensuing struggle for survival, the dispossessed and often hungry group moves off, sometimes to find new and unclaimed land, but more often to wrest it from another, preferably weaker tribe.

The seasonal migrations of the Eurasian tribes were dictated by the need for grass, for in summer the parched vegetation of the plain in the Asiatic sector of the steppe drove the tribes up into the lower mountain slopes, which had been rendered fertile by a heavier rainfall. However, in the autumn, the sharp cold withered the vegetation of the higher altitudes, and the tribes returned once more to the plain, which was by then again covered in greenery. In southern Russia, the general flatness of the steppe, the absence of harsh extremes of temperature and the smallness of the population enabled the nomads to establish camps for long periods on end, but in the extremes of winter and summer many of the tribesmen were inclined to move to the river beds where water was within immediate reach. The comparative easiness of life in the European sector proved irresistibly attractive to the Asiatic nomads, who were all too often tempted to trespass in the more clement southern and western portions of the steppe. Their eruptions were frequently no more than rapid raids into neighbouring ground, but some/ times a stronger tribe would intrude with the intention of gain/ ing a foothold in the more productive zone, and it often succeeded in displacing a weaker community. If the operation resulted in victory for the aggressors, most of the vanquished were generally killed, the few to escape death becoming slaves. Besides serving their conquerors, the survivors were also expected to adopt their masters' customs and beliefs, but the dispossessed often contrived to cling to their own traditions with such tenacity that, eventually, certain features from their own culture survived to blend with those of the conquerors. As a result, the combined outlook gradually came to be shared by the descendents of both until they were in their turn destroyed or assimilated by a new stream of invaders. It is in part because of this that it is so very difficult to define the exact racial links which existed among the tribes of the Eurasian plain, or even to distinguish the contribution made by each of them in form/ ing the animal art which is associated with the Scythians.

During most of the first millennium B.C. existence within the steppe was in the main tranquil, for the migratory movement which brought the Scythians to southern Russia evolved so slowly that the lives of the tribesmen underwent only a very gradual change. The mixed economy which they had estab/ lished as the basis of their life depended upon a certain degree of stability and, throughout the seventh and sixth centuries, the major wars in which the Scythians were concerned affected the warriors from only a section of the people. Most of the tribes/ men who had settled in the Kuban and in southern Russia continued to live the life of a pastoral people, with many of the men mainly occupied in caring for their flocks, in pursuing their favourite occupations of hunting, fowling and fishing and in maintaining trade with the Pontic Greeks.

The Scythians were polygamists, the sons often inheriting their father's wives, though at any rate one of these had generally to die at her husband's death that she might accompany him to the next world. In contrast to what has been observed in the Scythian burials, at Pazirik the women who died with their husbands often shared their coffins. This could be taken as an indication that the men there were monogamous or that the woman was a wife rather than a concubine.[1] The ancient Greeks' impression that Scythia was a matriarchy is not supported by archæological evidence; the idea was probably derived from the legends connecting the Amazons with Scythia. In fact, however, all existing material tends to show that although Scythian women were even more colourfully dressed than the men, they were nevertheless held in subservience, forced to travel in waggons with their children instead of riding beside their husband, obliged to devote themselves wholly to domestic pursuits and in some cases compelled to die with their consort. Nor were any emblems of authority placed beside them in their burial chambers.

The waggons in which the women and children travelled had trom four to six wheels. They were covered with felt roofs and the space inside was divided into two or three compartments or cubicles. Little clay models of these prototypes of the modern caravan have been found in some of the Scythian burials, one of the most interesting coming from near the Ulski barrow in the Kuban.[2] Strangely similar terra-cotta models of the same type have been found in the Pontus and in Cappadocia. Rostovtzeff ascribes the resemblance[3] to a community of race rather than to the influence of trade. The likeness is very surprising, for it is no less difficult to see how the Scythian examples could have been influenced by peoples living on the far shore of the Euxine than it is to account for the spontaneous development of the form along well-nigh identical lines. Yet so little is known about these remote days that some unrecorded migration may well have been responsible for the resemblance.

At this distance of time it is impossible to determine whether the covered waggons served the Scythians as permanent homes to which the men—who invariably moved about on horseback —returned at nightfall, as to a house; or whether the super-structures could be lifted off and erected in the camp much as a tent would be; or again, whether the Scythians habitually used tents, living in the covered waggons only whilst on the move. The decoration of the burial chambers at Pazirik tends to confirm this last suggestion, for it was clearly designed to transform the tomb into a tent. However, this conclusion need not necessarily hold good for the Scythians who were established in the European steppe, though they might well at one time have shared the simpler customs of the Altaians. But of one thing we can be sure: whatever their dwelling, whether waggon or tent, it is certain to have been comfortable and colourful. Furnishings discovered at Pazirik, corroborated by evidence from the Royal Scythian tombs and confirmed by discoveries in Bactria and at Noin Ula in northern Mongolia, show that the tribesmen possessed both felt- and wool-pile carpets. The painted decorations of some of the Crimean burial chambers and fragments found *in situ* at Pazirik show the use to which they put them. In addition to carpets, fabrics were widely used as tapestries and also, as at Pazirik, as hangings of religious import. From Pazirik too we learn that felt hangings decorated with elaborate appliqué designs were in general use, at any rate in the Altai.

Although the Royal Scyths favoured hereditary succession to the chieftainship, the kindred tribes seem to have preferred to elect their leaders. At Pazirik the exceptional tallness of the dead chieftains may be taken as an indication that the tribesmen

Plate 30

considered physical no less than intellectual pre-eminence a necessary qualification for the office. In the Kuban, as in the rest of the European section of the steppe, there is no evidence to show the way in which the chieftainship was obtained, but it is probable that, as in many other nomadic communities, valour carried some weight in the choice, riches following upon the high office rather than being the means to obtain it. This would help to explain the scene which is frequently represented in Scythian art, occurring in objects found in the Taman

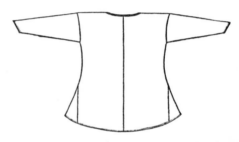

Fig. 4. Pattern of a shirt from Mound 2, Pazirik. V c. B.C.

peninsula, at Kul Oba, Voronezh and in numerous other burials, where the Great Goddess, whom the Scythians worshipped with particular fervour, is often shown seated on a throne whilst a nomad chief stands before her either to receive her approbation to his election or else to be invested by her with additional powers likely to prove helpful to him in his high office. The most impressive rendering of this scene of initiation or anointment appears on a felt hanging found in Mound 5 at Pazirik. There the Great Goddess is shown seated in majesty on a throne with a standard or sceptre set in her left hand, whilst a mounted warrior faces her with all the self-assurance of an elect being.

Everyday life was comparatively luxurious for the freeborn Scythian. The country as a whole abounded in fish and game, and in normal times the tribesmen were never short of food.

Plate 30

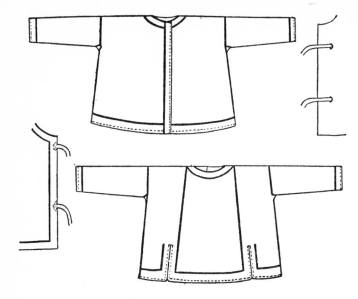

Fig. 5. Pattern of a jerkin from Mound 3, Pazirik. V c. B.C.

Their staple diet consisted of kumis, a form of fermented mare's milk which is still popular in the Caucasus and Mongolia, a good deal of cheese, and at times vegetables such as onions, garlic and beans. They could supplement this fare at will with tunny and sturgeon, and with every sort of game, as well as with horse-meat, lamb and goat. They often cooked their meat as a stew in a great cauldron of a shape peculiarly their own, but sometimes they turned it into a sort of haggis, which could presumably be transported. Like most tribesmen, the Scythians enjoyed good living. Hippocrates wrote that they were fat, lazy and humorous, and they would make the most of the passing hour, drinking wine, pledging brotherhood from a single vessel or loving cup, and indulging in singing and dancing to the accompaniment of drums and stringed instruments resembling lutes.

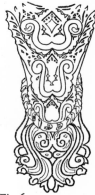

Fig. 6.
Trimming on a woman's stocking from Mound 2, Pazirik. V c. B.C.

The Scythians were also very fond of gay trimmings to their clothes. They could produce appliqué work of such delicacy and elaboration that it resembled the most accomplished embroidery. They made splendid but essentially practical garments for themselves, often using fur and leather. Indeed, their skins and hides were cured with such skill that they found purchasers far afield. The most lucrative fur markets were situated in Assyria, Bactria and Greece, in contrast to the meat, grain and slave markets which lay close at hand, for the most part in the Pontic region.

The skin and leather found at Pazirik is of the finest quality, varying in texture from very thick, heavy leather, through many gradations, to skins as fine and flexible as many a present-day product. Various items of clothing were unearthed there, many of which were in excellent condition. No trousers were found with any of the outfits with which the dead were provided for

Fig. 4   use in the next world, but two tailored woollen tunics survived in good condition. Both were skilfully shaped at the waist and flared at the hips by means of triangular insertions. These tunics

Fig. 5   were worn like shirts beneath jackets or jerkins. Three of these jerkins were preserved at Pazirik. They all followed much the same pattern, being straighter and somewhat longer than the shirts, but equally well tailored and smartly finished off with neat stitching, and then covered with ornate and spirited appliqué designs. One jerkin was of leather lined with sable, another was of unlined leather and the third of felt; all had straight hems, whereas the Scythian warriors represented on the carvings of the Hall of Xerxes at Persepolis are wearing garments shaped very like the modern tail-coat, thus bearing a closer resemblance to the coats which Radlov found at Katanda than to those discovered at Pazirik.4

All the clothes found at Pazirik amaze by the lavishness of their trimmings. In one instance profusely ornamented white

Fig. 6   stockings were mounted onto leather soles, the underneaths of which were as heavily worked as the uppers, for these became visible when the wearer sat cross-legged on the ground. Over-boots were adorned with an all-over pattern obtained by the juxtaposition of fur strips dyed in various colours. Two male head-dresses were also embellished with trimmings. In one the decoration took the form of a curious wooden castellation sewn to the crown of the hood. It is tempting to regard this as a badge of office or rank, some sort of crown in fact.

The women's clothes from Pazirik are even more ornate than the men's. A great cloak was unearthed there, cone-shaped and sleeveless, but with arm-holes cut in it. The garment was made of felt edged with fur, the whole of its surface practically covered in appliqué designs of an extremely intricate character. The robe worn with it was long and close fitting, with long straight sleeves and a tight-fitting bodice. Once again, both the sleeves and the front of the bodice were smothered in trimming. No women's head-dresses were found at Pazirik, with the

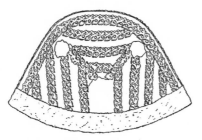

Fig. 7. Woman's cloak from Mound 2, Pazirik. V c. B.C.

exception of a long veil and a wooden cap with a plait of hair attached to it, but there was a profusion of belts, bags and satchels, many of which were trimmed with fur whilst others were decorated with applied designs. Some had a cord to pull them shut, others a handle or flap.

No complete garment of any sort has so far been found in any Scythian burial from the European area to show the exact way

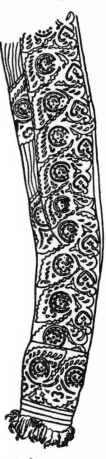

Fig. 8.
Sleeve from a woman's dress from Mound 2, Pazirik. V c. B.C.

Fig. 10

E

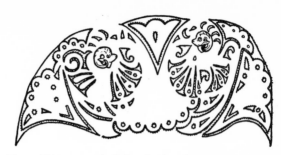

Fig. 9. Trimming on the bodice of a dress from Mound 2, Pazirik.
V c. B.C. About 7½ in. wide.

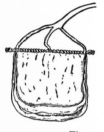

Fig. 10.
Leather bag from
Mound 2, Pazirik.
V c. B.C. Width,
10 in.

Fig. 11, Plate 4

in which the nomads dressed, but several of the finest gold vessels discovered in the richest tombs, though of Greek workmanship, are adorned with spirited scenes drawn from Scythian life. They are rendered with such obvious fidelity to detail that from the start they have been accepted by scholars as reliable period documents, which indicate the nature of the Scythians' dress and manners, as well as their physical appearance. The recent discoveries at Pazirik show how well justified these assumptions were as regards the general cut and trimming of the clothes reproduced on such objects as the famous silver vase from Voronezh and the electrum vessel from Kul Oba. In both cases the costumes are well-nigh identical with the actual garments preserved at Pazirik. The Voronezh and Kul Oba vessels date from the fourth century B.C., the garments may perhaps be slightly earlier in date.

On the Voronezh vase the main decoration shows a Scythian camp at rest, perhaps on the eve of battle. The scene unfolds as on a frieze, running round the bulge of the vessel. First we are shown the Scythian commanders assembled at a conference; next an experienced fighter advises a younger one on the use of his bow, and finally, warriors are shown preparing for the fray. In the Kul Oba vase the battle has been fought or is still in progress, and we see a chief listening to a messenger, a

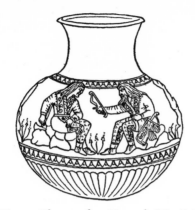

Fig. 11. Silver vase from Voronezh. IV c. B.C.

warrior tending the leg of a hurt companion, and another
dressing a mouth wound. In each case the comfortable, close-
fitting, belted tunics cut somewhat longer at the back than in
front are very clearly shown, as are the close-fitting trousers
heavily trimmed and tucked into soft, high boots. On the heads
peaked hoods are worn tied under the chin. The same type of
headgear is still in use, at any rate among children, in parts of
Russia today, where it is known as a bashlyk. All these features
closely correspond with actual garments found at Pazirik as
well as with the Persian representations of Scythians in the
great frieze of tribute bearers and prisoners at Persepolis. In
a figurine from Kul Oba a somewhat different costume is
reproduced, for there a bare-headed man is shown enveloped in
a garment resembling a bath robe. He clutches a cup in one hand
and a quiver in the other. Such robes may perhaps have been
worn by those participating in religious ceremonies or by
priests.

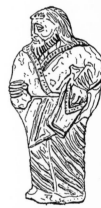

Fig. 12.
Hollow gold figure of
a man, possibly a
priest, holding a cup
and quiver. From Kul
Oba. IV c. B.C.
About 5 in. high.

Women seldom appear on metal-work of the Scythian period
and we know much less about their everyday clothes. They

seem to have worn long robes and high head-dresses covered with a veil. The similarity between the men's clothes represented on the Voronezh and Kul Oba vessels and the actual garments found in the graves at Pazirik, and the discovery in Mound 2 at Pazirik of fragments of a woman's head veil seem to justify the view that Scythian women dressed in very much the same manner as did those of Pazirik. Rostovtzeff believed that Scythian queens and princesses acted as priestesses to the Great Goddess and that they adopted special costumes when performing their religious rites. According to him they also wore them in death,[5] but apart from the discovery in certain of the more splendid women's burials from southern Russia of costume plaques bearing representations of the Great Goddess, there is nothing to show what the vestments were like, nor has anything been found at Pazirik that could throw light on this point. The most important examples of the Great Goddess plaques come from burials at Karagodenashkh and the Great Blisnitza or Twin barrows.

Fig. 49

In southern Russia and the Crimea some of the mounds have a rough and uncouth stone human figure set on their summits. The figures generally represent women, though a man is sometimes found among them, and centuries ago, the local inhabitants called them 'stone dames'—*kamenniya babi*. Early travellers associated the statues with the people buried in the barrows beneath them, but the opinion of scholars remains divided on this point. The dresses shown on them do not correspond with any of the garments found at Pazirik. Van le Coq[6] noticed that some had suspenders attached to their belts to hold up their soft high boots. The only other place in which he found similar suspenders was on the frescoes in the temples of early medieval date at Bazaklik in Turkestan, where they were worn by tall, red-haired, blue-eyed people whose faces were pronouncedly European. The statues of the women show high hats somewhat similar in shape to those worn by Welsh women of the eighteenth century, but a transparent veil covers them, thus further complicating the issue, for the shape of the hats makes it difficult to feel that the statues are connected with the Scythians buried beneath them, but the veils seem to imply the reverse. The majority of the figures appear to post-date the Scythian period by at least several centuries.

It is very probable that the Scythians evolved the style of their upper garment from the Assyrian tunic, but they soon turned it into a garb admirably suited to their equestrian form of life. There was then nothing in their costume that was likely to hamper their movements or to hinder them even when at full gallop on the fiercest steed. The close-fitting, swathed tunic and firmly tied hood also ensured excellent protection in all weathers. A variant of this costume was worn by all the horsemen of the Eurasian plain. It was the very antithesis of the swirling draperies of Greece or Rome, but the advantages which it conferred on mounted warriors were constantly being proved in battle. Yet the costume was never adopted by the Greeks and it was not until about 300 B.C. that the conservative Chinese were finally convinced of its benefits. At that date they were being harassed by the turbulent Hiung-nu, and they realized that without cavalry units it would be impossible to resist, still less to pursue and chastise the enemy. The decision to include mounted troops in the army could not be implemented without the introduction of reforms in military dress, for the traditional flowing robes and tight shoes worn by the Chinese were completely unsuitable for the new generation of cavalrymen. In their place the Emperor initiated the introduction of a costume modelled on that of his nomad enemies, and the baggy trousers and close-fitting tunics which survived as the national dress of China until the last war represented an oriental, yet clearly recognizable variant of Scythian dress.

If the Scythians were not the first to domesticate the horse, HORSEMANSHIP they were among the earliest, if not the first, of the central Asian people to learn to ride it. Both in China and in India, and possibly also in Egypt, horses had been used in the second millennium as beasts of burden for transporting loads, or for dragging carts mounted on solid wheels hewn out of stones or tree trunks; fighting steeds had also been trained to pull light chariots in battle, and at the chase. But the Scythians' success in war was largely due to the advantage which their mounted soldiers enjoyed over their foot enemies, a superiority which the latter were quick to appreciate. In consequence, almost im- mediately following upon the Scythian penetration into Asia, the technique of riding was suddenly mastered throughout the entire Middle Eastern area. Indeed, the rapidity with which foot soldiers were turned into cavalrymen was so great and so universal that it is quite possible that the horsemen who appeared in central Europe at much the same time had learnt to ride from their eastern neighbours. They, in their turn, trans- mitted the accomplishment to those living farther to the west. The Scythians used their horses only for riding, whether in war- fare or for hunting, regarding them as a means of rapid trans- port, and they continued to employ oxen for domestic purposes and for heavy work. In the Altai on the other hand, horses were used to pull the covered waggons in which the women and children were transported from place to place, as well as to drag the rough carts employed for such tasks as the transport of the heavy loads of great stones required for topping the burial mounds.

All the Pazirik tombs contained horse burials, the number varying from seven in Mound 3 to fourteen in some of the others. The animals were those which had belonged to the dead lord in the course of his life and they included his outworn mounts, and those he was using at the time of his death, as well as some two- and three-year-olds which he had probably selected for his future use.[7] Although professor Vitt[8] has established that the bulk of the ponies used at Pazirik were of wild Mongolian stock of Przewalski descent, and thus similar to those in use throughout Scythia, each Pazirik burial contained as well at least one thoroughbred of real quality, a horse of the much prized Ferghana breed. Stallions of this breed were coveted by the emperors of China, for they were so swift that the Chinese believed that they were of supernatural descent.[9] Vitt thinks that the Altaians must have obtained the stud animals by loot or as a form of tribute, but Rudenko is convinced that the horses found in the tombs had been bred locally. They averaged fifteen hands in height, and the majority were bays or chestnuts. Vitt is of the opinion that the hooves of horses of these colours stand up better to hard and rough ground than do those of paler coated animals.[10] The feet of some of the finest horses buried at Pazirik showed that they had spent the winter under cover, and there was evidence that they had been fed on grain, though the rough Mongol ponies lying in the same graves had been short of food prior to their death. The more valuable horses had had their ears branded, and all of them were geldings. In Scythia too all the riding horses had been gelded, and indeed the custom survived among certain Cossack communities in the Caucasus and central Russia until the revolution, where none but the very poorest would consent to be seen riding an ungelded horse.

At Pazirik every nomad had at least one horse and generally a good many more, and even the women were each provided in their tombs with a mount, though there is nothing to show the use they made of it during life. The cut of their dresses makes it seem unlikely that they had actually ridden. In Scythia most of the warriors owned a fair number of horses and the tribal chiefs generally possessed large herds of stallions and brood mares. The best herds were probably to be found in the Kuban and on the Dniepr, for the number of horses interred in the more important mounds in these regions often runs into hundreds. In the Poltava and Kiev districts on the other hand, it is rare to find more than one horse to a burial. The animals

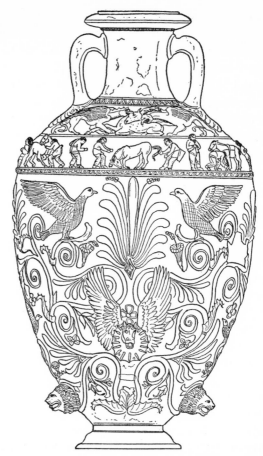

*Fig. 13. Electrum kumis jug from Chertomlyk. IV c. B.C.
Height, 27½ in.*

may have been harder to come by there, or the population may have been poorer, or again, the paucity of horses in a burial may be an indication that the inhabitants had developed a more advanced form of agriculture than that which was practised in the south, and that they preferred to spend a monotonous existence in wattle houses rather than continue to

live the exciting but precarious life of pastoral nomads. In the
Scythian burials which have been examined in Hungary it is
rare to find more than two horses lying in a tomb, and one
horse is more usual.

All the riding horses which were found at Pazirik had had
their manes trimmed, and the same practice must have been

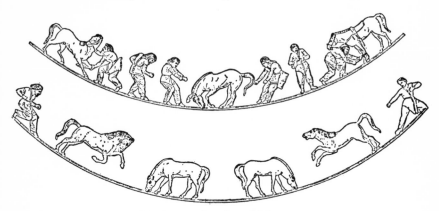

Fig. 14. Detail of the frieze on the Chertomlyk kumis jug.

followed in Scythia, for the manes are trimmed on the riding
horses represented on Scythian metal-work. The manes were
probably cut in order that they should not interfere with the
aim of a rider loosing his arrow at full gallop, for the cart-horses
which appear on the metal-work all have long, free-flowing
manes. Most of the horses had their tails plaited, but sometimes
they were knotted at half-length instead. A lively and convincing picture of Scythians at work on their horses survives for us
in the vivid decorations on a magnificent fourth-century electrum kumis jug from the Chertomlyk barrow. It is well over
two feet high and has two handles. It must have been made by
a Greek from one of the neighbouring Hellenic cities or by a
Thracian. The jug's base is decorated with a pattern of
acanthus leaves; above it, a frieze-like band unfolds to show

Figs. 13, 14

73

two young and two somewhat older Scythians catching ponies of the Mongolian type with a lasso. Some of the horses have their manes trimmed and are probably animals which had been turned out to grass after a period of service; the others have long manes and are obviously still unbroken, for they plunge wildly at the touch of the lasso. The scene is redolent of the steppe. It could have found its parallel in any Cossack community of pre-revolutionary days.

The Scythians owed much of their prowess in hunting and in battle to the superb skill with which they handled their mounts. But although they spent many hours schooling their animals, they must have devoted many more to fashioning their harness and their fighting and hunting equipment. All the horses' trappings which have so far been found, regardless of whether they come from the east or the west of the plain, reveal the great importance which the Scythians attached to the turn-out of their mounts. Can the inhabitants of England have inherited this outlook together with the decorative elements which affected 'Celtic' art?

HARNESS AND
EQUIPMENT

All the items of the nomads' harness which have been discovered in Eurasia are made with faultless skill from the finest materials available at the time, and all are adorned with a profusion of decoration that has not so far been equalled in any finds of a comparable character. At Pazirik the trappings are of breath-taking elaboration, yet the Altai was but a poor outpost of the Scythian world, and had similar pieces of harness survived in southern Russia, it is more than probable that they would have surpassed the eastern examples in intricacy and finish. Whenever comparisons between the two regions have proved possible, the pure Scythian work has shown a greater sophistication and a higher standard of workmanship, combined with a love of costlier materials. However, fate decreed that the non-perishable metal objects should be the ones to escape destruction in the European steppe, but that at Pazirik a great many materials which are usually the first to disintegrate should survive virtually undamaged for some two and a half millennia. Thus elaborately ornamented leather and felt saddles, saddle-cloths of felt and woven material, reins, bridles and bits have come down to us from Pazirik in excellent condi- tion. As a result, it has proved possible to reassemble the complete harness used by the horsemen of the first millennium and to estab- lish the exact manner in which their horses were caparisoned.

The portions of harness made from non-perishable materials, that is to say bits and metal cheek-pieces, are the same in the Altai as in the south of Russia, and this makes it seem probable that the pieces of equipment which perished in Scythia proper bore an equally close resemblance to the items which have survived at Pazirik.

The Scythians used a double curved bow made of horn and strung with sinews both for hunting and warfare. Their arrows had trefoil shaped heads, made, according to the phase of their development, either of stone, bone, bronze or iron. Bows and arrows were carried in a combined case known as a gorytus Plate 7 which was worn slung from the belt at the left hip. Both the Scythians and the Pazirik people shot over their left side in the Parthian manner.

In addition to their bows and arrows, the Scythians were equipped with swords which sometimes measured as much as two and a half feet in length. They also used short, double- sided daggers or akinæ, which they carried, rather as a Scot does his dirk, attached to their left leg by a strap, and in addition they employed deadly knives of varying lengths and different types, some having the incurving blades which are associated with China, others retaining European shapes. The celts, axes and picks which they used were similar to those which had been carried across Eurasia by the last European migration eastward. The Scythians also sometimes carried lances as well as standards surmounted by bronze images or heads of real or

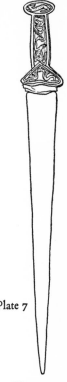

Fig. 15.
A sword from
Chertomlyk. IV c.
B.C. About 20 in.
long.

Plates 5, 6

75

imaginary animals. These poles may have had an heraldic significance, in which case their presence among the Scythians should be ascribed to Assyrian influence. With the passing years Assyrian and Persian elements tended to disappear, for the Royal Scyths were inclined to draw into increasingly close touch with the Greek outposts in the Pontus. So far as weapons were concerned, the Greek influence expressed itself in the adoption of shields and helms of Greek type, often even of Hellenic workmanship, and in the graves where the Greek influence is strongest, coats of mail also appear.

Plate 3

The Scythians excelled at lassoing, yet they preferred to pursue and shoot their quarry, and in the excitement of the chase they were very apt to forget whatever else they had on hand at the time. Thus, on one of the very rare occasions that a Scythian contingent had decided to engage in a skirmish with Darius and both armies had drawn up for the contest, the sudden appearance of a hare starting up between the enemy lines so completely distracted the tribesmen that, according to Herodotus, "immediately all the Scyths who saw it, rushed off in pursuit, with great confusion, and loud cries and shouts. Darius, hearing the noise, inquired the cause of it, and was told that the Scythians were all engaged in hunting a hare. On this he turned to those with whom he was wont to converse and said: 'Those men do indeed utterly despise us.' " The scene can readily be pictured, with the disciplined Persian troops stand-ing motionless awaiting the word of command, whilst the nomads rode helter-skelter after the one small creature streaking across the plain.

PHYSICAL
APPEARANCE

It is more difficult, however, to reconstruct the physical appearance of the Scythians than to understand their outlook. Were they short or tall? Long- or round-faced? Anthropological evidence is very meagre. The mummified remains found at Pazirik show that the chiefs were on the tall side, averaging 5 ft. 8 in., whilst the women were about 5 ft. 1 in. in height.[11]

Yet it is probable that these measurements held good only for the chieftains, since the tribesmen liked their leaders to be well built. The general average may well have been a good deal less.

The Scythians appear to have differed in appearance from the Pazirik people, for in their art they are represented as broad and squat. Yet there is no anthropological evidence to show what the Scythians were like, nor, conversely, have any pictorial representations of the people of Pazirik been found as yet, and the six mummified heads which were discovered in the mounds there are insufficient to fill the gap in our knowledge. Rudenko[12] has succeeded in establishing that the majority of the skulls found at Pazirik and at such allied burials as Shibe, Tuekt, Kurai and Katanda were European in type. This bears out Jettmar's view[13] that, at any rate until the fifth or fourth century B.C., the inhabitants of western Siberia were a fair-haired people of European origin, and that it was after that date that an influx of Mongoloids resulted in a very mixed type of population. At Pazirik the burials contained sub-brachy-cephalic, brachycephalic, mesocephalic and dolichocephalic skulls, which suggests a considerable admixture. From the representations on the Kul Oba, Chertomlyk and Voronezh vessels the Scythians seem to have resembled to a striking degree the peasants of pre-revolutionary Russia. Most scholars are, however convinced that no racial links exist between the Slavs and the Scythians, and Ripley[14] draws attention to the fact that in the central Russian burials of the stone age as many as three-quarters of the skulls were dolichocephalic, from the ninth to the thirteenth century only half belonged to this group, and after that date only forty per cent remained, the rest of the population being brachycephalic. Chvojka,[15] on the other hand, holds the view, which he reached as a result of numerous excavations conducted in the region, that the basic population remained the same from early to quite late times, but that the governing class changed both at each conquest and also with

Figs. 11, 13, 14,
Plate 4

the march of political events. The similarity in the appearance of the Scythians as revealed by the works of Greek metal/workers and that of the peasant population of pre/revolutionary central Russia might up to a point be fortuitous, resulting from the style of hair/cuts and the long beards favoured by both, but there are other resemblances which are harder to explain. The stocky build and large, rounded noses are thus common to both, and in addition, analogous traits are to be noted in the temperaments of both peoples. Both loved music and dancing; both were absorbed in art to the extent of enabling them to admire, assimilate, and refashion quite alien styles into some/thing entirely new and national; both had a talent for the graphic arts, and a well/nigh nation/wide preference for the colour red may also be noted. Again both peoples showed a readiness to adopt a scorched earth policy when invaded. Intermarriage may well have played its part in ensuring the survival in Russia of Scythian characteristics which continue to this day to find expression in the national outlook.

Another intriguing problem hinges on whether the Scythians wore beards. Some classical writers suggest that degeneracy and disease had made many of them beardless, but their repre/sentations on such comparatively late, yet first/hand documents as the Kul Oba, Chertomlyk and Voronezh vessels quite clearly indicates the contrary. The Pazirik excavations com/plicate the issue instead of elucidating it, for they show that whereas the majority of the tribesmen either plucked or shaved their faces, the Mongoloid chieftain who was buried in Mound 2, though by nature beardless, had been provided in his tomb with a sham beard, which was placed beneath his head/rest. It was made of real hair cut fairly short and dyed black, and was mounted onto a strip of leather, the ends of which met to tie at the back of his head. Furthermore a leather satchel containing additional supplies of black dye was laid beside this fake beard. It would seem then that the Pazirik people expected their chief

Fig. 3.

Figs. 11, 13, 14,
Plate 4

to appear in a beard at any rate on ceremonial occasions, and that, since this particular ruler, possibly because of his Mongol origin, may have been unable to grow one, he had to be pro- vided with a counterfeit which would enable him to appear correctly turned out in the next world. The similarity in the shape of his sham beard and that belonging to the robed man already referred to on page 67 is perhaps worth noting. In both cases the beards differ slightly in cut from those represented on the Kul Oba and Chertomlyk vessels, but if the suggestion be accepted that the robed figure represents a priest, the provision of a beard of similar shape in the tomb of the Mongol chief buried at Pazirik may indicate that this particular ruler played a no less important part in the religious life of his tribe than he did in its secular affairs. Or again, if the beard cannot be accepted as a symbol of office in either the political or religious field should it perhaps be regarded as a sign of rank or an emblem of cast, beards of this particular shape being worn by leaders whilst the ordinary freemen of the tribe, that is to say the warriors and hunters, had the pointed beards shown on the metal-work of the period?

Fig. 12

Herodotus noted that the Scythians did not use water for washing. Instead the women made an unguent of pounded cypress and cedar wood pulp, which they mixed with frankin- cense and water, rubbing the lot into a paste. They used this ointment as a cleansing compound, coating themselves with the substance and keeping it on for a day. Herodotus was surprised to find their skin beautifully clean and clear after they had removed it from their bodies.

Recent research has produced evidence to show that already by the fifth century B.C. some Scythians had established them- selves in southern Russia as settled agriculturalists. Spitzin tried to draw racial distinctions between those who had in- stalled themselves on the banks of the Dniepr and others who had settled in the districts of Kiev and Poltava.[16] But the

TOWNSHIPS

differences to which he draws attention are of a kind that must be due rather to the results of intermarriage with the local population than to any innate dissimilarity between the Scythians themselves.

Excavations conducted in the region of the Dniepr have disclosed the ruins of townlets which belonged to some of these Scythian settlers, or at any rate to some semi-Scythian communities. One of these, Kamenskoe,[17] can be taken as characteristic of this type of settlement. It is situated on the left bank of the Dniepr, practically opposite Nicopol. It was inhabited from the fifth to the second century B.C. and it covered an area of almost five square miles. From even a cursory examination of the site it becomes clear that already at this comparatively early date the Scythians were no mean builders, whilst its position so much to the north-west of southern Russia helps to account for the skilled construction of even the remoter Scythian burial chambers and to explain the ease with which the Christianized Russians were able to erect complicated churches of the Byzantine type virtually immediately after their conversion to the Greek Orthodox faith.

Kamenskoe was protected on three sides by natural defences formed of the steep banks of three rivers, the mighty Dniepr, the Korko and the larger Berezovka, but on the southern side, where the townlet lay exposed to the steppe, the inhabitants constructed a deep and most efficient earthen defence wall. This terminated at the south-west angle in a citadel. Immediately inside the wall a passage, varying in width from half to three-quarters of a mile, was kept as an open space. In peace-time it was used at night as a cattle pen, but in an emergency it was handed over to the town's defenders.

Inside this belt stood the houses. They were of three types. The most usual consisted of an oval central section built of wood, with outbuildings jutting out from either end. The more important were somewhat larger than the average, varying in size from forty to a hundred and seventy-six square yards. They contained two to three rooms, each leading into the other. The entrance to this type of house was always effected from the southern end, and the hearth was set either in the central or the northernmost room. The walls were of wood strengthened with an admixture of clay, with sloping roofs resting on wooden posts. Numerous bronze and iron tools, including quite a number of blacksmith's implements were found in them. The third type of dwelling closely resembled the latter both in plan and in the disposition of its rooms, but the structure was built wholly of clay. The only dressed stone found on the site was discovered on what the excavators assume to be the town's acropolis, but if this is indeed the case, then it must point either to the predominance of a non-Scythic, temple-worshipping element in the population or to a marked difference between the religious customs of the settled and those of the nomadic Scyths; the latter do not appear ever to have had or to have desired a shrine or permanent places of worship.

The inhabitants of Kamenskoe were poor, far poorer than most of the nomadic Scyths, but it is very probable that the settlers, irrespective of their origin, were mulcted of much of their wealth by their nomadic overlords. At any rate no important work of art, no notable piece of jewellery, and no magnificent domestic utensil has as yet been found in any urban Scythian site other than a necropolis.

The most impressive Scythian city which has been excavated up to the present time is that of Neapolis.[18] It lies on the outskirts of Simferopol, in the Crimea, and excavations were begun there in 1945 by Schultz and Golovkina. The town served as the capital of the Royal Scyths from the turn of the fourth century B.C. to the beginning of the Christian era. Though it is of comparatively late date, from early in the third century it already covered some forty acres of ground. It was at about this time that a great stone wall was erected round it to serve as a defence against the ever more menacing Sarmatian attacks. The wall varied in thickness from nine yards to about fourteen. It was pierced by a large gate flanked by defence towers. Within lay the capital of King Scylurus and his son and heir, the future King Palakus. It contained a number of impressive public buildings constructed of stone and roofed with tiles. They were adorned with elegant columns, ornate capitals and bronze and marble statues, the fragments of which still litter the site to serve as testimony of its former magnificence. Two busts—tentatively identified as heads of Scylurus and Palakus—reflect a new naturalism, which should perhaps be ascribed to the influence of Rome.

The residential quarter lay to the north of the town. There too the houses were of stone, and some idea of the appearance of the finest buildings can perhaps be obtained by recalling that the façade of the house which King Scyles had secretly acquired three centuries earlier at Olbia was adorned with figures of sphinxes and griffins. At Neapolis the better houses consisted of several rooms. They were built round a courtyard and their walls were decorated with mural paintings. Some of their storerooms still contained supplies of wheat, barley and millet. There is ample evidence to show that the life of the city followed an essentially urban pattern. Craftsmen and tradesmen of many sorts were established there. At least one potter had his own kiln, but many of the amphoræ found in the larger houses contained wines which had been imported from as far afield as Rhodes, Cnidus, Cos and Sinop. Trade must have flourished at Neapolis and the standard of living, at any rate among the welltodo, seems to have been high. Bones of horses, cows, goats and sheep were found in all quarters of the town in immense numbers, but those of boars and beavers were scarcely less numerous. The excavators interpret this as an indication that the hunting of game still continued to play an important part in the economy of the urban Scythians, though an elaborate agricultural system quite obviously now served as its basis.

Neapolis had large burial grounds. In the bigger necropolis, among a variety of tombs rich in gold objects, the excavators came upon an elegant and sophisticated, though strongly hellenistic, mausoleum belonging to a Scythian queen. A town as complex as this, with tombs as elegant, cannot have been of mushroom growth, for both features point to a fairly well evolved maturity, a stable economy and a broad outlook on life.

Although towns such as Neapolis or the smaller and poorer Kamenskoe were rare in Scythia, what towns there were shared in the life of the nomads, taking intense delight in it. Indeed, the urban Scyths, not altogether unlike the nineteenth-century gentry in England, retained their roots in the country and always kept their love of country pursuits alive. But the civilization which the nomads had evolved was as much in need of the cities that provided the skilled jewellers as the urban artists were in need of the steppe dwellers' inspiration, for Scythian art retained the direct, if complicated, outlook of those who live in the open-air. It was the nomads and not the townsmen who evolved its canons. The Scythians were not primarily sensualists; rather were they realists for whom the abstract and the sinuous had an irresistible appeal.

INTELLECTUAL AND ARTISTIC OUTLOOK

That they might have been no less fascinated by speculative thought, had they been given the opportunity to indulge in it, is shown by the life of Prince Anacharsis, brother of King Saulius, who was sent to Athens, where many of the policemen were Scythians, as ambassador. No sooner had he reached his post in 589 B.C., than he began to frequent the society of Solon and his circle of philosphers. Within a short time Anacharsis had forsaken politics to spend several years in searching for wisdom and divine truth. The Greeks held him in affection and called him 'Scythian eloquence', yet, eventually, the ambassador was obliged to set out for his own land. He travelled by a devious route, visiting as many countries as possible on his way, with a view to adding to his knowledge of the world. At Cyzicus his curiosity led him to agree to take part in the Eleusinian mysteries and he was induced to promise to give thanks to the Goddess of Cyzicus should he return to his native land in safety. Back at his brother's headquarters, he crept away one day with the intention of fulfilling his vow, but he was observed and his defection was hurriedly reported to the king. Saulius went in person to verify the report. Seeing his brother engrossed in alien devotions, he aimed an arrow at him, killing him outright. So perished Scythia's only philosopher, one whom even the Greeks had considered a sage, dying before his influence had made itself felt among his people.

Yet for all their savagery in warfare, for all their dislike of rhetoric and foreign customs, the Scythians were not boors. Their discernment in the artistic field and their love of domestic amenities is reflected in all their possessions. As with all nomads, the number of these had perforce to be strictly limited, yet the range and variety of the objects with which they surrounded themselves is truly amazing. No less astonishing is the care and skill which they lavished on making even the most trifling article. Practically every surviving example of Scythian work shows quality and the finest objects are truly magnificent. Apart from such essential items as arms and saddlery, and such primary necessities as clothes and coverings, the profusion of domestic utensils is as unexpected as is the variety of materials combined in the making of each individual article.

The pottery stands alone as being somewhat unambitious, but again it is found mainly in the poorest graves, for there was considerable disparity of wealth among the tribesmen. The local ware is coarse in texture, dull in colour, being either black, grey or buff, and primitive in shape, mainly taking the form of pots and only very occasionally, bowls. When pottery appears in the richer burials, it is always a high quality import from the Pontic colonies or from Ionia, and not the indigenous ware.

Like all primitive peoples, the Scythians were exceedingly superstitious. They believed in witchcraft, magic and the power of amulets. Their soothsayers foretold the future by means of bundles of twigs and by splitting bast fibres in much the same way as did certain groups of Germans in the Middle Ages. The most highly honoured of the Scythian magicians came from certain specific families. They spoke with high-pitched voices and wore women's clothes. They were probably eunuchs, but the Scythians believed that they had been afflicted with these feminine characteristics as a punishment for having offended against the Great Goddess by plundering her shrine at Ascalon. Their profession was not without grave danger, for a false diviner could expect no mercy. When proved wrong, though his women-folk were generally spared, he and all his male relatives were placed on a cart loaded with brushwood and put to death by burning.

SORCERY

The Scythians worshipped the elements. Their main devotions were paid to the Great Goddess, Tabiti-Vesta, the Goddess of Fire and perhaps also of beasts. She alone figures in their art, presiding at the taking of oaths, administering communion or anointing chieftains. Rostovtzeff[19] found that she had been worshipped in southern Russia long before the Scythians appeared there. Pottery statuettes of her were common in the Bronze Age in the country lying between the Urals and the Dniepr, even more along the Bug and Donetz rivers. There is a marked resemblance between these little figures and those representing the same deity in Elam, Babylonia and Egypt made centuries earlier. In the Crimea, the Great Goddess is not found much before the ninth century B.C., when she is depicted standing, holding a child in her arms, though she did not then represent the goddess of fertility any more than she ever personified a matriarchy to the Scythians. The latter

RELIGION

considered her as their political guardian, and Strabo noted that her cult was especially widespread along the Caucasian coast where she protected the seafaring tribes whom the Greeks thought of as the Argonauts. These people, and the Scyths of the Taman peninsula in particular, intensely resented the intrusion of strangers on their shores and they made a point of sacrificing to the Great Goddess all the Ionian sailors whom they succeeded in capturing. In Scythian art she sometimes appears as half-woman half-serpent, sometimes standing, sometimes seated between her sacred beasts, the raven and dog,[20] or sometimes with an attendant or in conversation with a chieftain.

Fig. 16

Plate 30

The Scythians also worshipped Papeus-Jupiter, the god of air, Apia-Fellus, goddess of the earth, Oetosyrus-Apollo, god of the sun and Artimpaasa, the celestial Venus, goddess of the moon. In addition, the Royal Scyths venerated Thamumasa-das-Neptune, god of water, and Herodotus thought that they sacrificed cattle and one prisoner out of every hundred captured to Mars and Hercules. Herodotus was surprised by the absence of images, altars and temples among the Scythians, and indeed, except for modest acropoleis of late date in Scythian towns, no places of worship nor any objects which can be definitely associated with religious ceremonials have so far been discovered. He was thus probably correct in thinking that the Scythians would forgather for worship at a specified spot, and depart from it after having performed their rites, without feeling that the ceremony had in any way sanctified the place in which it had been performed. In this they seem to have followed an Iranian tradition.

In place of temples and shrines the Scythians lavished all the veneration of which they were capable on the tombs of their dead, resembling the Chinese in their readiness to sacrifice their lives in safeguarding these burials. Yet all their care and vigilance failed to preserve their tombs from desecration by robbers, who, in almost every instance, penetrated into the barrows quite soon after the burials had taken place, rifling the contents with such thoroughness that hardly a single tomb has survived intact.

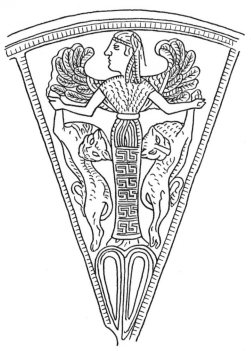

Fig. 16. The Great Goddess flanked by attendant beasts. Detail from the gilt and engraved silver mirror from Kelermes in the Kuban. VII–VI c. B.C.

Their burial rite was both elaborate and of extreme solemnity. In the Altai the interments seem to have taken place during only two seasons of the year, the spring and autumn, thus coinciding with the tribes' seasonal migrations in search of fresh grass. The habit of postponing burial made embalming essential, and Herodotus' detailed description of the process

BURIAL RITES

87

followed by the Scythians has been confirmed by the embalmed bodies discovered in the frozen tombs at Pazirik.

First the body had to be internally cleansed, stuffed with aromatic herbs, and sewn together. When all was ready the body was placed on a cart and the tribe as a whole, after cropping their ears and hair, followed the corpse with shouts and wails, slashing their arms and thrusting arrows through their left hands as the procession proceeded from village to village, until the whole of the dead man's territory had been visited. The journey had to last for forty days; only then could the body be brought back to the burial place. With a man of humbler rank the final progress, though still lasting for the prescribed period, was confined to visits to his relations and friends. When these had been performed the burial service could commence. The body with its supporting mattress was lifted from the cart and lowered into the burial chamber, where

Plates 5, 6

a bier sometimes awaited it. Standards surmounted by bronze animals were occasionally inserted cornerwise at the extremities of the bier, but sometimes poles surmounted by bells were

Plate 8, *Fig. 17*

placed there instead, for rattles of this sort helped to frighten the evil spirits away.

The dead chief was accompanied on his last journey by one of his wives, his head servants such as his cup-bearer, cook and head groom, and the horses which he had personally used in the course of his life. All were apparelled in their best clothes and finest jewellery, and each had a separate chamber or compartment allotted to him in the tomb. The master lay alone, with the most essential of his possessions close beside him. These consisted of his gold cups, his amphoræ filled with wine and oil, and his great cauldron filled with meat for his journey. His attendants and companions were each placed close to him, but his horses lay outside the burial chamber, yet within easy reach of it and under cover of the same mound, thus ensuring that they too would be close at hand on his awakening. All were splendidly caparisoned. After the tomb had been sealed, but before the erection of the mound, a wake was held above the burial chamber.

Up to this point Herodotus' account of a Scythian burial has been proved by excavations to be wholly reliable; he then went on to relate that it was customary, on the first anniversary

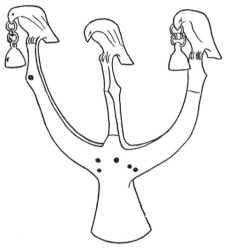

Fig. 17. Bronze rattle from Alexandropol. IV c. B.C.

of a chief's death, for fifty men from the dead ruler's bodyguard each—like every other member of his staff—a freeborn Scyth, and mounted on a splendid horse, to be killed. Their bodies were then cleansed and stuffed in the usual manner and the dead horses, each fully bridled and saddled, were impaled on stakes placed in a circle round the barrow. A dead rider was hoisted on to the back of each horse, and men and mounts were then abandoned to disintegrate as they stood guard over the tomb. No trace of this last grim ritual has survived, but it is hardly likely to have done so, since the bones of the dead would quickly have been picked bare by the carrion birds and the skeletons would have fallen to dust long before our day. Although it is difficult to believe that the Scythians can have been as wasteful of human lives as this custom demanded, Herodotus has been proved substantially correct in so much else that there seems little reason to doubt his accuracy here. But if such large-scale sacrifices were indeed made, they can surely have occurred only at the death of a king of outstanding importance.

According to Herodotus, all those who had taken part in a burial had to undergo purification. He tells us that this consisted in first soaping the body with a cleansing unguent, then 'they act as follows: they make a booth by fixing in the ground three sticks and over them woollen felts, which they arrange to fit as close as possible; inside the booth a dish is placed upon the ground, into which they put a number of red hot stones, ... and creeping under the felt coverings, throw some hemp seed upon the red hot stones; immediately it smokes, and gives out such vapours as no Grecian vapour bath can exceed; the Scyths delighted, shout for joy.'

Until 1929 no particular importance was attached to this description, but in that year precisely such stands (though some had as many as six poles) with their felt or leather sheets still stretched over them, a cauldron containing stones and hemp seeds standing within, were discovered at Pazirik. Each of the burials was provided with an outfit, the double burials containing two, one being for the man's use, the other for his wife. There, it was evident, the smoking or inhaling was not intended as an act of purification, but rather as a relaxation, perhaps serving to transport the smoker into an ecstasy similar to that attained by the use of certain narcotics. Probably the same was often true of southern Russia, where the habit was likely to have been regularly indulged in.

Sources

Numbers in parentheses refer to the Bibliography on p. 201.

1   Rudenko (92), p. 254, disagrees with this view.
2   For an illustration see Minns (18), pp. 50⁄1.
3   Rostovtzeff (27), pp. 11 and 224.
4   Radlov (47), Vol. II, p. 144.
5   Rostovtzeff (27), p. 73.
6   Van le Coq (36), p. 88. For an illustration of a 'stone dame' see Minns (18), p. 239, fig. 149.
7   Rudenko (92), p. 148.
8   Vitt (96), pp. 163⁄205.
9   Yetts (39), p. 231, and Llewellyn, p. 39.
10   Rudenko (92), p. 71.
11   *Ibid.,* p. 67.
12   *Ibid.,* p. 62.
13   Jettmar (44), p. 519.
14   Ripley (25), p. 354.
15   Chvojka (76), Pt. I, pp. 172⁄90.
16   Spitzin (94), No. 65, pp. 87⁄8.
17   Grakov (80).
18   Piotrovsky, Schultze and Golovkina (67), pp. 69⁄103. For illustration of busts see p. 72, fig. 17.
19   Rostovtzeff (70).
20   Rostovtzeff (27); for illustrations see Plate 23, 5.

CHAPTER III

The Tombs

ALTHOUGH PRACTICALLY ALL the Scythian tombs which have been excavated had been rifled in antiquity, they have nevertheless disclosed to us a wholly unexpected world of complex imagery and solid achievement, whose exis‑ tence had not even been hinted at by any of the surviving ancient texts.

The Scythians, as we learn from their own proud and defiant retort to the taunts of Darius, valued their burial grounds above all their possessions, venerating them with a passion that was perhaps increased by their lack of temples and holy sites. To them the burial ceremony was an intensely mystical and august ritual, but it was also a singularly costly affair, not only in labour, material and worldly goods, but also in life. The loss in horses was especially high. Recent discoveries show that orthopædically faulty animals were sometimes killed off in Hungary[1] and a proportion of those buried in Altaian graves suffered from similar defects,[2] but many of the horses found at Pazirik were in excellent condition at the time of their death. Information on this point is lacking with regard to the Kuban and south Russian burials, but the numbers of horses killed at important funerals in the Kuban was tremendous. There the figures varied from a score to several hundred, the highest to be recorded being at Ulski, where some four hundred had been buried.

The most important and impressive of the Scythian burials are the royal tombs of southern Russia, and of them all Chertomlyk is perhaps the richest, both in the variety and artistic quality of the objects found in it and also in the well‑nigh fabulous intrinsic value of the gold‑work. Like so many other burials, Chertomlyk had attracted the attention of thieves, but in this instance a fall of earth in the entrance shaft they had dug trapped and killed at any rate one of the gang, leaving the objects he had amassed piled up in a corner of the tomb. Since this robber was unlikely to have dug the trench single-handed, it is probable that his companions escaped with some of the booty. Nevertheless, the archæologists who opened the tomb some two thousand years later still found in it much that was of considerable monetary value and a great deal more that was of absorbing interest.

The barrow was unusually elaborate in plan, for it contained a central burial chamber with four minor ones radiating from it. The first chamber to be entered by the excavators contained a small Scythian cauldron, a magnificent gorytus complete with arrows, and five knives with bone handles and iron blades. In the main chamber they found fragments of a carpet, but these were too decayed to give any idea of its pattern. Hooks for clothes to hang on were still in place on the walls and ceilings, but the garments which had once hung there had perished, and only the stamped gold plaques with which they had been trimmed lay in heaps where they had fallen to the ground. Placed in niches set at floor level in the walls were further personal belongings and some gold vases. In the north-eastern chamber stood six amphoræ still holding the dregs of the wine and oil that had once filled them and also a bronze mirror mounted on an ivory handle.

The dead man lay on his back, facing east. The setting in which he took leave of this world was of extraordinary opulence. A fine bronze torque encircled his neck, a gold ear-ring had been placed in one ear and there were gold rings on all his fingers. According to custom, an ivory-handled knife lay within easy reach of his left hand, together with a gorytus containing sixty-seven bronze arrow-heads and an ivory-handled riding whip laced with gold. Fragments of an ivory casket, a silver spoon, numerous gold plaques from his clothes, pendants, gold tubes, beads and buttons were also found here. In the third small chamber lay two bodies, each adorned with a gold torque, gold bracelets and rings, and a belt decorated with gold plaques, together with the gold plaques which had trimmed the clothing strewn about their bare bones. Beside them stood a bronze cup, a silver ewer, a gorytus containing arrows, and a whip. In the fourth chamber were fragments of a bronze bier that had once been decorated with an elaborate

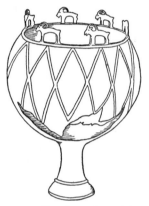

Fig. 18. Bronze cauldron from Chertomlyk. IV c. B.C.

design carried out in dark and light blue, green and yellow paint. A woman's body lay on it, still wreathed in gold bracelets, fingerrings and earrings. Twentynine stamped gold plaques, twenty gold roundels and seven gold buttons lay intermingled with her bones. On her head were the remnants of a purple veil with the fiftyseven gold plaques which had formed its trimming still in place. Within her reach was a bronze mirror set in blue paste. Nearby lay a man's body, probably an attendant's, with a bronze bracelet on his arm, his knife and arrowheads within grasp of his left hand. Between the bodies stood an elaborately ornamented silver dish, and it was there

that the famous Chertomlyk vessel itself was found. A large
bronze cauldron, measuring three feet in height, with six
splendidly modelled goats ranged round its rim to serve as
handles, was also found in the tomb, as well as a smaller bronze
cauldron, numerous minor objects in gold, a great ornamented
sheet of gold which had been ripped off the king's gorytus, five
splendid swords, and numerous fragments of delicate Greek
pottery. Ten horses lay fully caparisoned outside the burial
chamber, but in the same compound. The trappings of five
were embellished with gold decorations, those of the rest with
silver.

Figs. 13, 14
Fig. 18

Plate 7
Figs. 15, 19

The construction of an important burial place required much
effort. First a clearing had to be made in the steppe, next a
sloping trench of varying length was dug and at its far end a
shaft, often of impressive dimensions, had to be sunk in the
virgin soil. Great wooden props were used to strengthen the
sides. Then the trench had to be transformed into a corridor by
means of a conically-shaped roof and the shaft turned into a
chamber by the erection above it of a gabled roof set on massive
posts resembling columns.

Once the structure had been completed, its decoration was
begun. In southern Russia, the walls of the main chamber were
hung either with wicker or rush matting, birch bark, thatch or
rugs, whilst at Pazirik felt was used. At Karagodenashkh in
the Kuban, on the other hand, frescoes were preferred, and the
figure of a deer at pasture was still visible to the excavators who
uncovered the burial. The ceilings of the main chambers
generally received the same treatment as the walls, thus giving
the effect of a chamber or tent, or possibly even the cubicle in
the covered waggon in which the defunct had spent many of
his living hours. Within this chamber a smaller, roofed construction or tabernacle was often erected to shelter the body. In
the sixth century B.C. in southern Russia, this inner structure
often seems to have followed the lines of the outer chamber, but

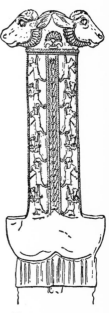

Fig. 19.
Hilt of the king's
golden sword from
the Chertomlyk
burial. IV c. B.C.
About 6 in. long.

two centuries later a dressed stone construction, ascribed by Rostovtzeff to Greek influence,[3] surmounted by a wooden roof, was at times preferred. The body was placed on a mattress and laid in this inner chamber, often resting on a bier covered with a fabric or a mattress of its own. Sometimes the bier was replaced by a coffin, which was generally either embellished with a painted design or decorated with an ornamentation in gold. Adjoining the main chamber were the side chambers, built for the dead man's servants and close attendants. The number of these substructures varied from one, as at Krasno-kutsk, to two, as at Tsymbalka, and to as many as four at Chertomlyk and Alexandropol. The attendants were generally buried in the western chamber, the grooms receiving prefer-ential treatment. Thus, at Chertomlyk, they alone of all the retainers lay in comparative isolation beneath a roofing of tree trunks, whilst the five others were placed with their feet point-ing towards their masters, so that, at their awakening, they would rise instantly to face him.

Most of the Royal Scythian tombs are situated close to Alexandropol and Nicopol, but some have also been found on the fringe of the Greek settlements of Panticapæum. The most notable of the Alexandropol-Nicopol groups are the Tolstiya Mogily or Big Barrows, which vary in height from 30 to 70 feet and in circumference from 400 to 1200 feet or so, with the burial chambers measuring from 9 ft. 6 in. to 15 feet in length and 7 feet in width. These chambers were often sunk as much as 42 feet below virgin soil. The Panti-capæum barrows are no less impressive, and include such rich and famous mounds as Altin Oba (Golden Barrow), Kul Oba (Mound of Ashes) and Tsarsky or Royal Barrow. Of them all only Altin Oba had escaped the attention of robbers, possibly because its burial chamber was built of enormous blocks of dressed stone, set to overlap each other so as to meet in the centre in an impressive pointed vault. The conception is surprisingly reminiscent of Mycenæan constructions and Minns is surely correct in thinking that the Scythian chiefs buried in this type of tomb found Hellenic culture so much to their taste that they employed Greek masons to build their sepulchres for them.[4] Indeed, nothing could have been easier than to engage Greek workmen either at Tsarsky Kurgan, which lay very close to the Greek colony at Kerch, or at Kul Oba, which was only four miles to the west of it, or at Altin Oba, which was equally close at hand.

The mound which was raised over Tsarsky Kurgan is one of the biggest, measuring 55 feet in height and 820 feet in circumference, but although that of Kul Oba was somewhat smaller and rather more oval in shape, it concealed a rather larger chamber, measuring 15 feet by 14 feet and 17 feet high. Here the king lay alone in the main chamber, his body resting in a coffin which had been made of either juniper or cypress wood and lined with a veneer of ivory engraved by a superb Greek artist with a beautiful scene of the Judgment of Paris. He wore a felt cap on his head decorated with strips of embossed gold. Encircling his arms were inch-wide gold bracelets with magnificent terminal figures, in the one case of Peleus and Thetis, in the other of Eos and Memnon. Electrum bracelets with sphinx terminals were clasped round his wrists. They were of the finest Greek workmanship, and so too were the electrum amulets which had been attached to his clothes. By his side lay a great Scythian sword, two and a half feet long, its blade three and a half inches wide. Its sheath was decorated with gold designs of great beauty. A cauldron containing meat stood close by. Four statuettes were found by the body. All are of particular interest on account of being worked in the round instead of being stamped out in the customary manner. One is of special importance for it shows two Scyths drinking brotherhood from a single cup.[5] Numerous gold plaques were discovered beneath the dead man's head and Minns noted

that some of them must have been made from the same
stamps as those used for producing identical plaques found at
Chertomlyk, Ogüz and The Seven Brothers barrows.[6] This
form of mass production suggests that there must have existed
recognized workshops, or at any rate some noted jewellers, who
worked permanently in one place, using moulds of such infinite
delicacy that the finished plaques look as though they had each
been laboriously hand produced. The Hermitage Museum's
collection of Scythian plaques numbers over ten thousand, but
although the smaller ones were quite often repeated in large
numbers, it is rare to find the bigger ones (which seldom
measure more than an inch across) showing the same design.
Plaques of the same type were found by Griaznov in 1927 at
Shibe, sewn to the clothes of an old man of Mongoloid type,
but only silver ones have so far been discovered at Pazirik.

In the main Kul Oba burial a narrow, box-like partition
separated the king's body from his weapons and arrow-heads.
In another, somewhat similar compartment stood a wooden
bier mounted on turned legs on which lay the body of a
woman. Her attendant was placed at right angles to her in yet
another compartment. The woman wore an electrum diadem on
her head, a gold necklace of great beauty encircled her neck and
precious rings were on her fingers. Her arms were decked with
bracelets, and at her waist were two large medallions, somewhat
surprisingly decorated with the head of Athena. There were
also three smaller medallions, all of which Minns thinks must
originally have belonged to a Greek temple. Between the
woman's knees reposed the famous Kul Oba vase. A mirror
lay beside her. Like much of her jewellery, it was of Greek
workmanship, but it was mounted on a Scythian handle.
Scythian also were the long knife and five somewhat shorter
ivory-handled ones belonging to her attendants. From Kul
Oba too comes the famous gold figure of a recumbent stag
which probably served as the centre-piece of a shield. Though

Plate 4

Plate 24

æsthetically less satisfying than the splendid example from Kostromskaya, it must, nevertheless, rank with the master-pieces of the metalworker's art.

It is thus evident that when the Scythians were at the height of their prosperity, that is to say from perhaps as early as the

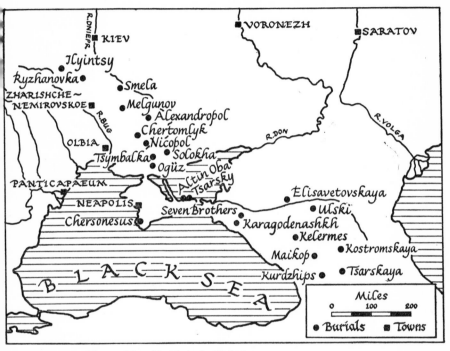

Fig. 20. Map of burials in the Black Sea area.

seventh century to as late as the fourth or third centuries B.C., a Scythian king and queen and the great chieftains of the land were buried in their finest clothes and jewels, and they were often provided with additional clothes for use beyond the grave. They also invariably took with them their sacred gold and silver vases, rhytons and drinking cups. Amphoræ filled with wine and oil, a great bronze cauldron containing supplies of meat and their essential weapons were placed close at hand. The head servants, likewise wearing their best clothes and with their weapons within reach, but with bronze jewellery instead of golden, lay in simpler chambers. The dead man's wife was, however, always provided with a tomb scarcely less sumptuous than that of her husband, and sometimes a male attendant, possibly her groom, was chosen to accompany her. All the bodies were laid on their backs, facing east.

In the richest funerals the chieftain's body was generally conveyed to the grave on a waggon drawn by at least two horses, more usually by four and sometimes by as many as six. Less important people were laid on mattresses placed on a bier and they were carried in procession by members of their households. In each case the funerals must have been noisy affairs. At the head came standard-bearers carrying poles surmounted by

Plates 5, 6

bronze or iron representations of fierce-looking birds or stately beasts. They were followed by a group of tribesmen swirling

Fig. 17

huge metal rattles and shaking bells fixed to wooden handles, who accompanied their flourishes with piercing shrieks designed to frighten away the evil spirits. Next came the funeral waggon or the carried bier, the horses adding to the noise with the jingling of their harness bells. On either side of the body walked men carrying a canopy surmounted at each corner by an

Plate 8

heraldic-looking bronze beast and hung with still more bells. Then followed those who were to die at the grave that they might accompany their master to the world beyond, and the procession closed with the rest of the tribe howling and wailing as they followed behind.

These proceedings bring to mind the ritual followed in China under the Han emperors, and it is thus not surprising

Fig. 21

to find that it was also in force at Pazirik. There, however, no heraldic-looking standards and no rattles or bells have as yet been discovered, though certain local features, which will be described later in this chapter, give these burials a unique

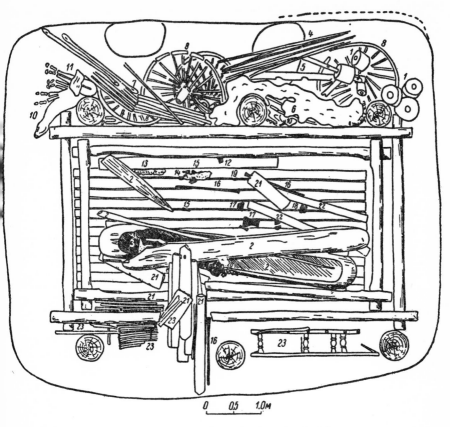

Fig. 21. Plan of the burial at Mound 5, Pazirik.

1. *Waggon wheels.*
2. *Coffins and their lids.*
3. *Bones of the dead.*
4. *Waggon pole.*
5. *Ladder.*
6. *The pile carpet described on page 141.*
7–9. *Waggon parts.*
10. *Bodies of dead horses.*
11. *Felt rug or hanging.*
12. *Sherds of pottery jug.*
13. *A goatskin.*
14. *A sheepskin.*
15. *Table legs.*
16. *Six wooden supports for the hemp-smoking tent.*
17. *Bone drum.*
18. *Felt cushion.*
19. *Domestic utensils.*
20. *Woman's head-dress.*
21. *Beams used for roofing the burial chamber.*
22. *Remainder of waggon parts.*
23. *Part of the cart.*

character, raising problems whose solution must still largely depend on the results of future excavations.

In southern Russia, once the body of the dead man had been placed in the burial chamber beneath a specially constructed tabernacle, and his possessions laid out beside him, his dead companions were disposed in the places which had been allocated to them. They had died either by poisoning or strang⁄ ling. The turn of the horses came next, all fully caparisoned in

Figs. 22 and 23

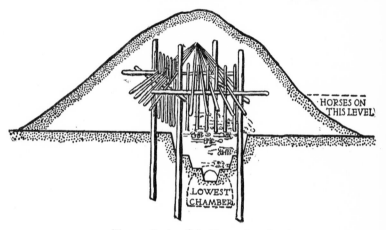

Fig. 22. Section of the Kostromskaya burial.

their finest harness. Each was killed by a blow delivered on the head. Their bodies were placed round the human tombs, the disposition varying in accordance with the space available for them. Whenever possible they were arranged in an orderly manner, either in rows or pairs, or even in a circle round the burials. Sometimes, however, some had to be buried at a higher level than that of the main tomb, but even then, the bodies were always put within the same burial shaft. A layer of earth was sprinkled over them and the funeral cart was then broken up and the fragments laid on this earth. Only then was the shaft filled in and the soil rammed down over the tomb. Sometimes

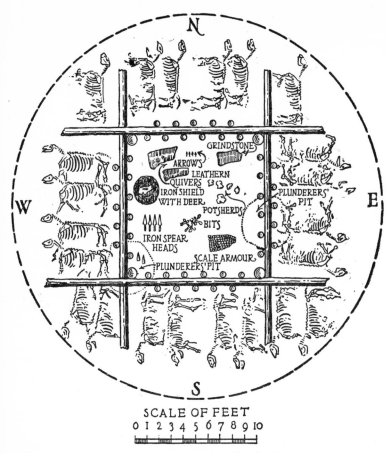

Fig. 23. Plan of the Kostromskaya burial.

a strengthening of stones was added. The wake was held at ground level, and not until the feast had been consumed was the final stage of the ceremony—that of constructing the mound embarked upon.

Such was the interment of a wealthy prince, the head of a powerful clan, the proud owner of numerous herds of cattle and valuable strings of horses, a chieftain with several wives, the

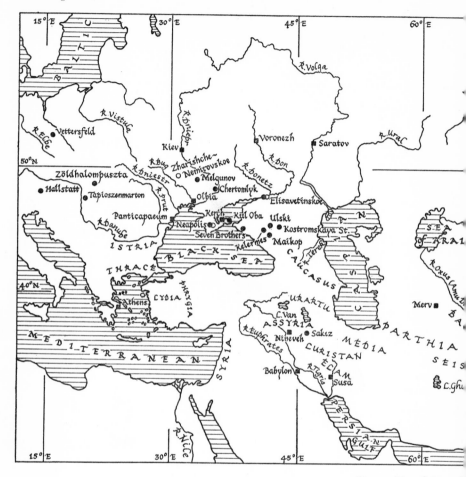

Fig. 24. Map of sites and

owner of a great deal of jewellery, much of it of gold. Less affluent chiefs, though still men to be reckoned with, were also buried with considerable magnificence. Instead of having a barrow to themselves, however, they usually reposed in the larger of two obviously related ones. Burials of this type are

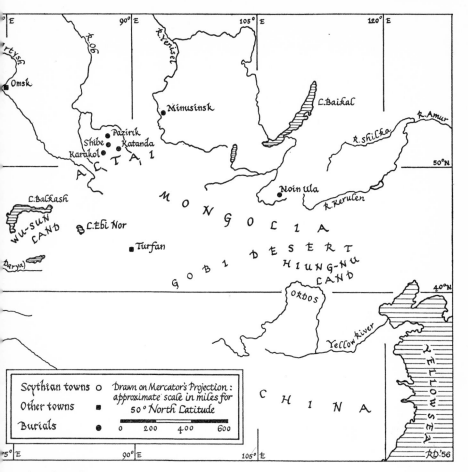

area of Scythian influence.

called Twin Barrows (*Blisnitzy*) in consequence. Such chieftains' barrows have rather steep sides, sometimes strengthened
by stones, and a flattened summit. Beneath is a single burial
chamber sheltering the body of the dead chieftain, his military
equipment, food and wine for his journey to the next world

and the best of his personal possessions. Among the latter, objects of Greek workmanship are often found. A man such as this was sent to the world beyond alone, unaccompanied by human attendants, but his horses followed him, their bodies generally forming a circle round the burial chamber. The smaller, round, companion mounds contain numerous poor burials. They probably belonged to the ordinary members of the tribe.

Before considering the more easterly burials, it may be convenient to glance at some of the Scythian burial grounds in northwest Russia, Prussia and the Balkans, all of which differ slightly from those of the Kuban, and very considerably from the royal tombs of southern Russia. Thus, in the rather more wooded districts of Kiev and Poltava, where the population consisted in the main of settlers, or at any rate of semisettled inhabitants, the Scythian barrows are smaller, averaging only some seven feet in height. Fewer horses were buried in them, and the contents are generally poorer, bone often replacing gold or other metals. Ornaments of wood were probably used there, but very few have withstood the rigours of the climate. Many of the tombs in this region date from the fourth century B.C., when the burial chambers were often given a surround of wooden posts that supported a flat wooden roof. Often such chambers were also provided with wooden sides or walls as well as with oak floors. Here too the dead man was always buried with his weapons, his gorytus, and sometimes with a coat of mail. The objects which were thought to be essential to him in the next world were also placed in the tomb. In most cases a mirror was included, and sometimes a few gold objects were added, but the number of horses killed seldom exceeded two.

Burials farther to the west are rare. An important find was, however, unearthed by a farmer's plough at Vettersfeld in Prussia. The collection of objects is puzzling. It consisted of a jar and the complete equipment of a Scythian warrior, but with no traces of horse bones. Especially outstanding was a shield, made of pale gold, with a centre-piece consisting of a remark-able figure of a fish. A breast-plate found with it is the only one of its kind associated with a Scythian. With it lay a panel of gold torn from a sword sheath worked in the Scythian style and a dagger with the characteristic Scytho-Siberian heart-shaped guard. No jewellery or horse-trappings were found with the hoard. It is dated to the early fifth century B.C. A somewhat similar, though less important find was made at Plohmühlen in Schleswig.[7] Neither of them helps to explain the presence of Scythian objects so far to the north-west of their homeland and it rests with future archæologists to establish whether the Scythians penetrated to Prussia in the form of single com-munities or as a group of considerable size, and whether they travelled in small batches by devious routes or whether a large concourse followed a definite road across Silesia.

In the fourth century B.C. the Royal Scyths of southern Russia attempted to shift their headquarters from the lower Dniepr to the north and west of their earlier centre. Shortly afterwards, the eastern fringe of the Balkans became a Scythian outpost, and as a result, the region contains quite a considerable number of Scythian burials. Bessarabia, Wallachia and the Dobrudja in particular retain important traces of their sojourn, and some of the graves there have yielded impressive examples of their artistry. In Romania the richest finds come from the Bukhovina where the most interesting mounds are to be found in the vicinity of Cuciurul Mare, Satu Mare and Boureni in Moldavia, but nowhere in the Balkans have the burials as yet received the detailed and systematic study which would enable comparisons to be drawn between the customs in force in these Scythian outposts and those adhered to in Scythia proper.

Some Scythians also penetrated into Hungary towards the year 500 B.C. They probably followed a route leading across Moldavia and Transylvania, for both districts are rich in

Plates 25, 28

mounds. Many of the objects found on Hungarian soil are of outstanding artistic importance. Foremost amongst them are the two magnificent gold stags which were discovered, the one at Tapioszentmarton, the other at Zoldhalompuszta. The number of Scythian burials in Hungary is very considerable and finds have often been unearthed by agricultural workers. Apart from chance discoveries of this sort, over eighty-five major burials had been scientifically excavated in the country up to 1939. All included horse bones, though the number of animals killed was invariably low and they were often of poor quality. The scientific information adduced from these excavations has, however, remained disappointingly small.

As we move back across Russia the picture becomes fuller again. To the east of the royal tombs, the tombs of the Kuban afford particularly rich and interesting examples of Scythian burials of early date. The Barrows of the Seven Brothers can be chosen as a characteristic example of the finer type of Kuban burial, though the objects found at Kelermes are perhaps of greater intrinsic value. In the Kuban Greek influence is less to the fore than in the royal tombs, and although examples of Greek workmanship occur in almost every burial, none gives the impression of having been expressly made for a special patron of the region or even for the Kuban in particular. Rather do the articles seem to be current Greek exports, chosen by the Kuban Scyths either because they corresponded well enough to their own local taste or because no others were available. Thus no vessels similar to the specially commissioned vases from Kul Oba, Chertomlyk or Voronezh exist in the Kuban, but instead the indigenous style is seen there at its most marked.

This style appears in its purest form in the horse-trappings and in many of the weapons, notably in the swords, daggers and knives used by the men. The jewellery is, however, apt to reflect Persian influence in very much the same way that the

personal adornments of the Royal Scyths were strongly affected
by Hellenic elements. A golden leopard from Kelermes, for
example, had its eye sockets and nostrils filled in with glass
paste and semi-precious stones, while its ears were encrusted
with that early form of cloisonné enamelling which shows
strong affinities with Achæmenid work of the eighth and
seventh centuries B.C. Another Kuban burial contained a gold
gorytus, a magnificent belt and a golden diadem surmounted
with griffins which bear a marked resemblance to certain of the
Oxus finds.

Plate 9

Local features are also to be noted in the construction of the
Kuban burial chambers. Thus at Kostromskaya, four vast
poles marked the corners of an area some 10 ft. 6 in. square.
Four beams were laid across them and six poles were then
placed on the inner side of the square and five others just outside it, but in the spaces between the inner poles. The tops of all
the poles were then drawn together to meet in the centre to
form a roof. Only twenty-two horses were buried in this mound
but in it was found an iron shield bearing as its centre-piece the
magnificent figure of a crouching stag made of gold which goes
by the name of the Kostromskaya stag.

Figs. 22 and 23

Plate 23

The numerous burials which have been opened in Siberia
present certain quite unique problems and two groups of tombs
are specially interesting. The earliest to be discovered were the
frozen burials of Katanda, near the river Berel, belonging to the
early iron age. These too had for the most part been looted in
antiquity and little gold remained in the tombs, though some
bronze objects had been left behind by the thieves. The larger
Katanda burial was covered by a cairn only seven feet high, but
it measured over a hundred feet in circumference. Horses had
been included in the burial, but Radlov did not specify their
number.[8] The burial chamber was fourteen feet square and it
had been roofed with larch and lined with birch bark. The
tomb lay beneath a stratum of ice. A bundle of clothes was found

preserved in it. It included a silk coat shaped like a modern tail-coat, lined with sable, edged with leather and trimmed with stamped gold plaques, a coat of ermine dyed red and green, and trimmed with gold buttons and gold plaques, an ermine tie and a silk band decorated with carved wood figures of horses, fabulous beasts, monsters, stags and bears disposed in a row. Some closely resemble certain animal forms found at Noin Ula in Mongolia. The human bodies rested on low wooden tables or stands and some other pieces of furniture recall examples from Pazirik.

Radlov excavated another group of frozen tombs on the banks of the same river, but at a point lying somewhat closer to Bukhtarna. There, the bodies of sixteen horses were found beneath a layer of wood, disposed in four rows, with their heads pointing to the east. All were fully caparisoned. Their bits were of iron and their leather bridles were adorned with ornaments of carved wood and birch bark covered with thin sheets of gold. Here the human burial chamber was situated at a slightly lower level. It contained a coffin made out of a hollowed tree trunk which was then adorned with copper birds closely resembling similar representations found in the Scythian tombs of the Volga and Ural regions. A man's body lay in it with the weapons similar to those belonging to a Scythian nomad placed within his reach. A mirror and a cauldron of the Scythian type were found in the chamber, but there was nothing in the tomb which could help towards assigning anything like an exact date to it.

In 1927 Rudenko and Griaznov were able to examine another group of tombs of much the same type. These were situated at Shibe close to the river Ursul. The largest of these mounds resembled the Pazirik burials. It measured some hundred and thirty feet in diameter, but once again the cairn was only about six feet high, and the burial chamber roughly twenty-one feet deep. The grave belonged to an old man. His body lay in a wooden coffin with a boy close beside him. The bodies of fourteen horses were placed in the northern portion of the tomb, but the burial had been rifled in antiquity and little of value was left in it. In 1934 Kiselev excavated another mound belonging to this group. It contained the body of an old man of Mongoloid type and a woman wrapped in a red silk shroud trimmed with gold plaques. She wore a gold diadem, and a mirror and various other valuable objects, all bearing a strong likeness to the Pazirik finds, were lying beside her. In 1950 further burials which closely resemble those of Pazirik were examined at Başadar, a site situated in the same locality. In this instance the body lay in a wooden coffin, the sides of which were decorated with a carved row of four tigers advancing from left to right. They reappear on the lid together with two stags, two wild boars and three mountain goats rendered in a some⁄ what more flexible style than that of Pazirik. Fourteen horses were interred in this burial which, notwithstanding the unusual character of the coffin,[9] must again have belonged to a tribe very similar to that of Pazirik.[10] An unusual find was that of a harp.

Indeed this whole series of burials so closely resembles the infinitely richer tombs excavated at Pazirik that both groups must have belonged to tribes which were either closely allied to each other or shared a similar culture, though the Pazirik people were wealthier and more powerful than the others. The burial ground at Pazirik is correspondingly larger, comprising some forty mounds. They vary in size as well as in shape. Six of the larger ones have so far been examined as well as some of the smaller ones. All are situated on an eastern slope of the Altai, at the level of the summer pasture land where the earth, though frozen in the winter, thaws out in the spring and summer. The ground is very rough, and even the largest mounds are low, being topped, like cairns, only with the earth dug out from the burial chambers and a covering of boulders. The size of the mound is thus determined by its circumference

Plate 10

PAZIRIK

rather than its height, the largest measuring from about 120 to 160 feet in diameter. Some of the smaller mounds are marked by an outer circle of stones instead of being topped with boulders, or again covered with stones placed to form sections of different patterns. No two of the Pazirik mounds are identical, yet all are allied to the same group of people. Nor are they all of precisely the same date. Of the larger mounds to have been excavated Mounds 1 and 2 belong to the second half of

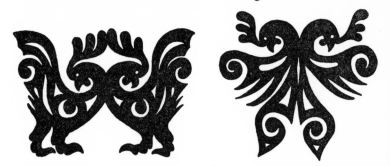

Fig. 25. Cut-out leather cock silhouettes from Mound 1, Pazirik. V c. B.C. About 6 in. high.

the fifth century B.C. and Mounds 3 and 4 to its last quarter; Mound 5 is to be assigned to the fifth-fourth century B.C. and Mound 6 to the first half of the fourth century B.C. It is possible that some of the smaller differences between the mounds may have in part arisen from intermarriage between the people of Pazirik and those from different tribes, with the result that their local customs underwent certain minor changes. In their broad lines, however, the burials are all of one type. In each case horses are found in the mounds, occupying a third of the entire burial space and invariably lying in a separate compartment situated at the northern extremity of the tomb. Lack of space often made it necessary for some of the horses to lie at a higher level than that of the main burial, but as far as possible their bodies were set out in an orderly manner.

Fig. 21

In the larger mounds, the burial chambers occupied some forty-five square yards. They were enclosed by double walls, the outer ones being made of rough logs whilst the inner ones were smoothed on the inside. The space between them was sometimes left empty, but at others it was filled in with brush-wood. The floors were generally smoothed over, but occasion-ally they were sprinkled with gravel. The ceilings were lined with birch bark, as in the Kuban and at Shibe, and then

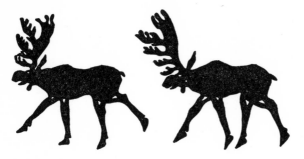

Fig. 26. Cut-out leather stag silhouettes from Mound 2, Pazirik. V c. B.C. About 6 x 7 in.

covered with a layer of twigs. The construction is very elaborate and goes to show that even in the Altai the nomads had acquired considerable skill in building in wood by as early as the fifth century B.C. The standard of domestic amenities must also have been high, for in all the Pazirik tombs which have so far been examined, the walls of the burial chambers had been lined with felt. It was held in place either by moulded copper nails or by wooden ones. Nails for the suspension of clothes and other articles were fixed to the walls. In Mound 2, the floor was covered with black felt. In Mound 1, the wall hangings were of surprising elaboration, for the dark brown ground was bordered with a band of white felt set between two strips of white, red, yellow and blue dog-tooth patterns, whilst the wide central band displayed a row of fierce and very spirited,

Fig. 64

Fig. 61

Figs. 25, 26

snub-nosed and snarling lions' heads executed in bright blue and red felt. The chamber of Mound 5 was also hung with felt. Though only fragments survived, the archæologists succeeded in reconstructing its design. The main motif consists of a large winged creature with a human head surmounting a lion's body. It was vividly coloured and set against an off-white ground bordered with brilliantly tinted birds enclosed in a scroll.

The Pazirik dead were laid in coffins hollowed out of vast larch trunks similar to those found at Shibe and Baṣadur. In each example the lower part of the coffin was somewhat deeper than the lid and, at Pazirik, contained two holes cut at each end to take either the ropes by which it was lowered into the grave or those by which it was carried. In Mounds 1 and 2 the rims of the coffins were decorated with beautiful silhouettes cut out of leather and then gilt, in the one case showing strongly stylized, confronted cocks, in the other a row of running deer.

The bodies which were found at Pazirik had been embalmed. Indeed, the practice of bi-annual burial adopted by the tribe made this a necessity—it was not just a luxury for the most distinguished chiefs. In contrast to the Scythian practice of laying the chief in a private chamber and placing his wife in an adjacent one, at Pazirik it was usual for the man and wife to share the same coffin, the man lying at the top end, the woman at the lower. Both were placed on their backs with their heads to the east. The bodies lay on rugs placed on large felt blankets, the edges of which overlapped sufficiently to fold across the bodies in order to shield them from the coffin lids. Again in contrast to Scythia, the Pazirik dead were placed in their coffins only partially clothed, that is to say with their coats slung over their shoulders and the women's bodices laid across their breasts. The men wore no trousers, and although a good deal of clothing has been recovered from the tombs no trousers have been found in any of the burials. The head-dresses were, however, placed on their heads and their feet were shod in stockings and shoes. The dead lay with their left hands resting on their breasts and their right on their pubis. Not much jewellery was found on them, probably because the thieves who had penetrated to the burial chambers had removed everything of value, but some silver amulets in the form of horses, silver belt buckles and silver and bronze costume plaques lay with the bones, together with an occasional ear, ring, a necklace or two, a few glass beads and the all-essential looking-glass.

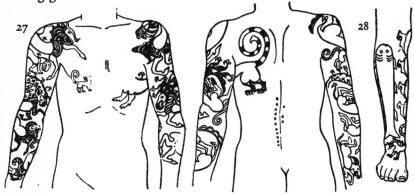

Fig. 27. Tattooings preserved on the body of the chieftain buried in Mound 2, Pazirik. V c. B.C.

Fig. 28. Tattooings on the leg of the chieftain.

Some of the most exciting discoveries were made in Mounds 2 and 5, where the bodies of two chiefs were found to have been covered in extremely intricate tattooings. One body had greatly deteriorated with the passage of time, but on the other, that of a man aged about sixty, beardless and of Mongoloid type, the very man in fact who had been provided with a sham beard, large sections of the design survived on his arms, chest and back. The man had died in battle. The designs tattooed on his body consisted of animal forms. They were essentially Scythian in style and motif, and so lively and spirited in conception and

Figs. 27, 28, 57–8

execution that they must rank with the finest drawings of the Scythian school. Their quality speaks for itself but their meaning remains obscure. Nothing has been found in any Scythian tomb to suggest that tattooing was common amongst the nomads of the European steppe. Hippocrates does refer to their custom of branding themselves for medicinal purposes, but he is unlikely to have confused tattooing with branding. The idea of tattooing themselves may have reached the Altaians from the esquimaux, who were in the habit of doing so, and who may have come in contact with the inhabitants of southern Siberia earlier than is thought. Or again, they may have learnt to tattoo from the people of the Punjab who, according to Frazer,[11] have long believed that, at death 'the little entire man or woman inside the mortal frame will go to heaven blazoned with the same tattooed patterns which adorned the body in life'. Since Przyluski[12] traces the cult of 'the Golden Stag' among the Salvas back to the Scythians there is no reason why the link between the two people should not have been a two-way one. Rudenko,[13] however, basing his view on statements of Herodotus, Hippocrates, Xenophon and Pomponius Mela, all of whom noted that tattooings served to indicate rank amongst certain Asiatic peoples, believes that they were used for the same purpose at Pazirik, yet among the Kirghiz it was, until fairly recently, reserved for the bravest among them. There was nothing in the Pazirik tombs to help solve the problem and nothing to link the sham beard with the tattooings; the dead man remains an enigmatic figure. His wife had the soft hair of a European, but she wore a wooden headgear with plaits attached to it, as strange as her husband's beard and tattooed decorations.

Although thieves had robbed the human graves at Pazirik, they had not penetrated into the horses' burial chambers, and in these everything was found undisturbed. As in the human graves, so in these all the walls were hung with felt which was just as elaborately worked as were the hangings in the human sections. Many of the horses had been in excellent condition at the time of their death. The best had been fed on grain which had probably been grown for the purpose in the plain during the spring months and carried up to the summer encampment. Its use as an animal food goes to show that the tribe had achieved a mixed economy of its own, abandoning its pastoral occupations during the spring months for agricultural pursuits. All the riding horses were chestnut or bay geldings, and many were well-bred animals, though some rough Mongol ponies were included in the burials. The condition of the feet of the finer ones suggests that they had been kept in stables for some time prior to their death.

Both in Scythia and at Pazirik the horses were buried fully caparisoned, all their accoutrements, including whips, being placed in the tomb. The opulence of the harness is quite astonishing. All of it is lavishly decorated, much of it with gold or bronze plaques, the rest in carved wood or birch bark, worked felt or fur, again enhanced with either gold or lead foil. Most of the Pazirik equipment has come down to us in excellent condition, thus making it possible to establish the exact way in which the nomads harnessed and turned out their mounts. This will be described in the next chapter, but here attention must be drawn to a curious, virtually unique trapping of so puzzling a character that even though no less than eight examples were found at Pazirik, their derivation and exact purpose cannot as yet be fully explained.

Fig. 39

These finds consist of eight horses' masks or rather headdresses, belonging to eight splendid Ferghana horses. The two masks found in Mound I completely covered the horses' heads, fitting right over them like veritable masks. The foundations were made of moulded leather which had then been covered with coloured leather of an infinitely finer texture. The masks were decorated, in the one instance with a scene of a panther

Plates 11, 12

attacking a stag, in the other of a horned and winged dragon attacking a griffin-like animal, which was in its turn about to pounce on a tiger. These scenes were carried out in bright blue and green fur. A row of cocks, shown in profile, were likewise made of coloured furs. In addition, both masks were profusely decorated with gilt, silvered and coloured leather roundels and crescents, and, strangest of all, both were surmounted by a pair of towering antlers, partially gilt.

The presence of antlers at first seemed to suggest that the masks were intended to disguise the horses as stags. As a result, the burials were thought to belong to an age when the stag, though no longer used as a means of transport, still remained associated with the burial ceremony, in which it may well once have taken the part that was filled by horses at Pazirik.[14] On these grounds it seemed as if the Pazirik people were passing through a period of transition, evolving from a 'stag' stage of culture to one dominated by the horse, and as a result the burials were tentatively dated to a very early period.

The following season's excavations led to the discovery, this time in Mound 2, of further examples of somewhat similar head-dresses. Although the majority were in bad condition, it proved possible to reconstruct one complete outfit, and it then became apparent that this example differed so considerably from the first two masks that it invalidated all the conclusions which had been based on them. To begin with, the new head-dress was not a mask in the real sense of the word, for it only partially covered the animal's head, coming down in a peak over its eyes and leaving the face exposed. It was thus more of a head-dress than a mask. It was made of white felt, shaped at the top as a hood, with the ear-flaps open in the front and the edge of the peak jutting out over the eyes trimmed with a row of gold animal figures. A felt boss set between the ears in the centre of the hood served as a mount or support for the leather head of a horned mountain goat. On the back of this creature's neck

Fig. 29

perched a bird made of white felt covered with leather, its gilt wings half raised, its cock's tail resplendently curved. Though this extraordinary, heraldic, aggressive composition defies explanation, it served to demolish the theory that the Pazirik people still adhered to the stag cult at the time of these burials.

Whilst drawing attention to the plumes with which the horses in the sculptures from Nineveh are decked, Rudenko[15]

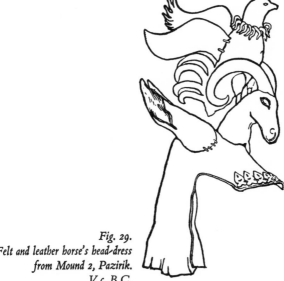

Fig. 29.
Felt and leather horse's head-dress
from Mound 2, Pazirik.
V c. B.C.

is nevertheless not inclined to ascribe the Pazirik head-dresses to Assyrian influence. Rather does he believe that in both instances the idea of adorning the heads of horses in some way was derived from a common source, probably of west-Asiatic origin and dating to the first quarter of the first millennium. The Assyrians developed the idea in the course of the seventh century, along the lines illustrated in sculptures at Nineveh. At a somewhat later date, the Altaians transformed the plumes into masks of the Pazirik type. Another somewhat similar instance is offered by the Torrs chamfrain discovered in Kirk-cudbrightshire[16] in 1829. Rudenko is convinced that the Pazirik examples were not reserved exclusively for use at burials, for one of the damaged masks showed signs of so much wear that it must have been used at numerous ceremonies before playing its final part in the Pazirik burial. The Pazirik head-dresses were worn in conjunction with boldly decorated leather sheaths covering the horses' manes and tails, the patterns on them being of a stylized character and formed either of cut-outs or of leather encrustations. Somewhat similar mane coverings can sometimes be seen on Assyrian sculptures.

Fig. 63

In connection with the head-dresses Kiselev[17] draws attention to four statuettes of horses which Radlov discovered at Katanda and to a fifth of much the same sort found in the neighbourhood. All five show a reclining creature with a griffin's head set upon a horse's body. Each one has four holes cut in the top of its head and Kiselev is convinced that in each case two of the holes were intended to serve as ear sockets, the ears being made of some different material from the body, whilst the other two were made to hold antlers. If this was so, and it seems most probable that Kiselev's surmise is the correct one, the explanation for the one group of finds would also hold good for the other.

The carts which were used at the burials were broken up and buried in the mounds at Pazirik just as they were in Scythia. At Pazirik most of the carts were primitive affairs. They were mounted on solid wheels hewn out of tree trunks and they had seen such heavy use that their wheels were badly worn. Rudenko thinks that they were used to transport the stones which were needed for topping the mounds and not, as in Scythia, for the body's final progress to the grave. A cart in Mound 5 was of a different type. It was an elegant and elaborate vehicle, mounted on four spoke wheels, each measuring almost

Fig. 30

six feet in diameter, but lacking the iron rim or tyre usually found on wheels of Scythian make. The cart was made of birch wood, some of which was turned and all of which could be dismantled and slung on pack animals for transporting across unsuitable ground. A raised, platform-like seat was provided for the driver and the entire superstructure was

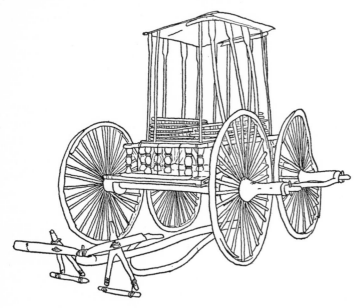

Fig. 30. Cart (capable of being dismantled) from Mound 5, Pazirik. V—IV c. B.C. Width, 10 ft.; height, 9 ft.; wheels about 6 ft. 6 in. in diameter. When assembled the parts were secured in position by straps.

covered with a black felt hood magnificently decorated with Chinese-looking swans executed in coloured felt cut-outs. The turned woodwork closely resembles the turned table-legs found in the Pazirik tombs. Both were assuredly produced locally, yet the cart is of a much more sophisticated type than any of those which have so far been discovered in the Eurasian plain.

It is thus tempting to associate this unusual carriage—as yet a unique example of its kind—with the country which inspired, or more probably which actually produced its hood, that is to say with China. Historical justification for the suggestion may be found in the Chinese chronicles, some of which record that the contemporary Emperors of China attempted to secure peace on their western boundaries by marrying off their unwanted princesses to the more turbulent of the neighbouring nomad chieftains. The unfortunate brides were each presented by the Emperors with a parting wedding present consisting of a cart requiring four horses to draw it, and they were then dispatched into the wilds, there to do their best for China and their uncouth husbands.

The woman lying at the chief's side, however, had the soft hair and the dolichocephalic skull of an Indo-European; it is therefore wiser to ascribe the cart to emulation, and not to think of her either as an exquisite exile from the refined and luxurious court of China who had withstood, and perhaps secretly come to delight in the rigours and unconventionality of a nomad's life, or as another princess Hsi-chün. This unlucky creature was married in about the year 110 B.C. to the central Asian chief K'un Mo, king of the Wu-sun. He was old and feeble, and they met on only very rare occasions over a cup of wine. She bewailed her loneliness in this sad little poem:

> My people have married me
> In a far corner of Earth:
> Sent me away to a strange land,
> To the king of the Wu-sun.
> A tent is my house,
> Of felt are my walls;
> Raw flesh my food

With mare's milk to drink.
Always thinking of my own country,
My heart sad within.
Would I were a yellow stork
And could fly to my own home.[18]

SOURCES

Numbers in parentheses refer to the Bibliography on p. 201.

1 Bökönyi (54), pp. 108–9.
2 Tsalkin (95), pp. 147–57.
3 Rostovtzeff (27), p. 47.
4 Minns (18), p. 194.
5 For illustration see *ibid.,* fig. 98, p. 203.
6 *Ibid.,* p. 204.
7 Martin (46), p. 11.
8 Radlov (47), pp. 106–9.
9 An unusual find consisted of a harp placed beside the mummified body of a woman, lying close to that of a mummified man.
10 Mongait (85), p. 148.
11 Frazer (12), p. 180.
12 J. Przyluski, 'Un ancien peuple du Penjab, Les Salva'. *Journal Asiatique,* vol. CCXIV, Paris 1929, p. 337.
13 Rudenko (92), pp. 140–1.
14 Mestchanínov (84), Nos. 1 and 2, p. 6; also Rudenko (92), p. 226; also Marr, N., USSR Academy of Science, 1929, No. 17, pp. 324–5.
15 Rudenko (92), p. 226.
16 Atkinson and Piggott (3), p. 197.
17 Kiselev (81), pp. 341–2.
18 Poem 53 from *170 Chinese poems,* translated by Arthur Waley.

CHAPTER IV

Worldly Goods

THE OBJECTS which have been discovered in the Scythian tombs of southern Russia and at Pazirik provide a fairly complete inventory of the articles in daily use among the nomads of Eurasia between the early seventh and about the second century B.C. In so far as their tools are concerned, we know from both Pazirik and southern Russia, as for instance from Smela in the district of Kiev, that they used narrow wooden spades, seldom measuring more than about four inches across, mounted on rounded handles varying in length from forty-six inches to about four feet. Wooden picks and celts were also found at Pazirik, with over a hundred wooden hammers and mallets. The latter were usually made of plane wood, and were heavy and massive, with an overall length of about sixteen inches, and handles ten inches long. Bone mattocks made of horn or tusk were also usual; they were mounted on wooden handles. Ladders took the form of poles with notches some two inches deep cut in them. Nails were made of wood as well as of moulded copper, and wooden pegs were universally used. Blacksmiths' tools included a wide variety of moulds for casting anything from arrow-heads, harness parts and sickles to personal adornments, amulets and domestic utensils. Vast cauldrons have been found, measuring as much as three feet in height and weighing anything up to seventy-five pounds and without a single flaw in their casting. Ploughs probably followed the lines of the Chinese models unearthed as far west in Siberia as Minussinsk, where they date from the fifth century B.C., and they bear the mark of a fish or a cross, or the laconic words 'made by man'. In the Yenissei, knives for working fur and leather have also been found, and similar implements were probably in use at much the same date at Pazirik.

AXES

Although Herodotus stressed the importance of axes in Scythian equipment, and although exquisitely made models executed in precious materials served the chiefs as symbols of authority, the number of both types actually discovered in the burials is far smaller than might have been expected. The simplest working axes had only a single loop, but double looped examples seem to have been equally common through/ out Eurasia. Most characteristic perhaps are those having a bronze cutting head with the opposite end terminating in an animal's head, but others had an iron head with a three/ pronged projection of considerable size on the non/cutting end. One of the finest symbolic axes came from Kelermes. The nomads generally wore a whetstone suspended from their belts. Many of these are mounted in gold settings decorated with floral or geometric motifs.

The knives they used varied in length, shape and material, and metal knives with straight handles encased in wooden sheaths are no less characteristic and no less numerous than crescent/shaped ones made either of bronze or iron, mounted in ivory, wood or bone. Maces are comparatively rare, and although some lathes have been found which were used for turning birch and plane wood, their number remains small. Stone files, on the other hand, are found in profusion.

ARMS

When the trefoil/shaped arrow/heads were made of iron they were generally cast. In the Altai the shafts on which they were mounted were decorated with highly stylized snake or feather designs executed in black or red paint. The bows were

Plate 7

strung with sinews and carried with their arrows in a gorytus; this was generally made of a wooden foundation encased in a covering of precious metal or leather decorated with stamped designs of the utmost delicacy and elaboration. The patterns range from zoomorphic designs to geometric forms. Hunters frequently used a lasso made of sinews, whilst warriors usually

Figs. 15, 19

carried a sword. These generally followed a Persian shape, and their handles were intricately ornamented with Persian designs, though they often terminated with the figure or head of an animal of Scythian character. According to date, the blades were either of bronze or of iron, but the sheaths were generally encased by thin sheets of gold, delicately embossed and often inlaid with ivory, paste or precious stones. The scabbards were provided with a hook for fixing the chains or straps which held them to the wearers' belts. Daggers or akinæ were given a heart-shaped guard and were likewise Persian in inspiration. Spears and javelins were used only occasionally, but many warriors wore a sort of shirt made of metal scales and adorned with a pectoral ornament. In the earlier examples the scales were of bronze; later, iron was used in preference. In either case, the metal shirt was mounted on a red felt lining. A helm was made on the same principle as the shirt and was similarly mounted on felt, but with the passing centuries the more markedly hellenized chiefs preferred to substitute Greek helmets and breast-plates for their native scale armour, and some even added a Greek greave to the outfit.

Plate 13

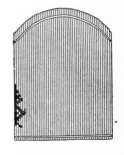

Fig. 31.
Shield from Mound
3, Pazirik. V c. B.C
Height, 2 ft. 3 in.

The Scythians usually carried round shields when they rode to battle. These seldom exceeded fifteen inches in diameter and were small enough not to hinder the rider. They were adorned with a centre-piece of the finest workmanship, usually an animal, which was often executed in gold and sometimes embellished with inlay and jewels. At Pazirik the shields were completely different, yet they closely resembled those shown in the hands of the Scythian warriors portrayed on a magnificent gold comb found in the Solokha burial of central Russia. Thus instead of a circular disc, the Pazirik warriors carried a shield made of a framework of wood, covered with leather, rectangular at the base and rounded at the top. As a further contrast, the Pazirik shields were completely plain and are thus to be numbered with the very few objects which the nomads did not attempt to decorate. Apart from their asymetrically-shaped

Plates 9, 23–5

Fig. 31

bows, their arrows and daggers, no other weapons were
found at Pazirik so that it is not yet known to what extent the
military equipment of the Altaians resembled that of the
Scythians.

SADDLERY   Both in Scythia and at Pazirik, the native, nomadic art is
seen at its purest in the horse-trappings, which are characterized
by a striking unity and a liveliness of compelling force. The

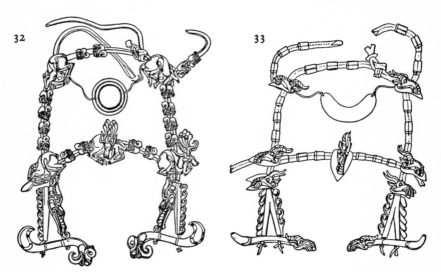

Fig. 32. Bridle from Mound 5, Pazirik. V—IV c. B.C.

Fig. 33. Bridle from Mound 5, Pazirik. V—IV c. B.C.

excellence of the craftsmanship and the quality of the designs
combine to produce some truly splendid objects. The in-
genuity and skill which went to the making of each bit of
harness is quite astonishing, but it is the Pazirik finds which
alone reveal the full extent to which the love of ornate trappings
governed the nomads. Although scenes such as those which
Figs. 13, 14   appear on the Chertomlyk vase and on other pieces of Scythian
metal-work throw considerable light on the way in which the

Scythians harnessed and decked their horses, and although archæological material from southern Russia has confirmed the conclusions derived from such representations, many technical details remained obscure. It was only when the Pazirik excava‐ tions had produced several complete sets of harness that the minor points were settled and the way in which the Altaians accoutred their riding horses became known. Comparisons between the bits and the nose and cheek pieces from Pazirik and those from the European section of the steppe show that

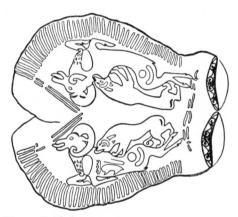

Fig. 35. Saddle from Mound 1, Pazirik. V—IV c. B.C.

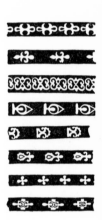

*Fig. 34.
Saddle‐straps with open‐work patterns from Mound 1, Pazirik. V c. B.C.*

these pieces were substantially identical throughout the entire region, and it therefore seems more than likely that the perish‐ able portions of the equipment, though they failed to survive in the west, were very similar to those which were preserved at Pazirik.

Both in the east and in the west of the plain the bit was a two‐ piece affair closely resembling the modern snaffle. At Pazirik the bridles consisted of nose, cheek and forehead straps as well as of an ear‐band, the whole being secured by a buckle placed on the left side of the animal's head. This halter‐like bridle had

Figs. 32, 33

I

been used in Assyria from as far back as the first half of the first millennium, and was probably much the same as that invented by the world's earliest riders. At Pazirik a metal plate, held in position by a leather strand, was placed in the centre of the horse's forehead. This plate, the cheek and nose pieces, and every point at which a strap intersected another, indeed, even the straps themselves, were all lavishly decorated with geometric patterns and animal shapes. These either perforated the straps or were applied to them in a variety of materials. All the straps

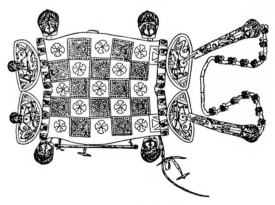

Fig. 36. Saddle from Mound 5, Pazirik. V—IV c. B.C.

were made of excellent leather, carefully worked, richly orna´ mented and often embellished with gold plaques or carvings covered in gold or lead foil. The buckles were of bone, the bits were for the most part of bronze or copper having a small admixture of lead, or again of wrought iron. They too were often given animal or floral terminals. Metal stirrups had not been invented at this date, but leather slings figure on the Chertomlyk vase.[1]

Figs. 34–7
Plate 14

The glittering effect created by the ornate bridle was sustained and enhanced by the colourful saddles and saddle´cloths. The saddles which are represented on Scythian metal´work seem closely to follow the lines of the actual saddles found at Pazirik. The latter were made of two felt cushions, varying in size from twenty to twenty-four inches in length. Some of the later examples were attached at the back and front to wooden saddle frames and both types were mounted on felt sweat-bands. Two straps were sewn to the back and front of each cushion and these, together with a central girth, breast-band and tail strap, served to keep the saddle in place. The cushions were stuffed with stag-hair, and they were often fitted

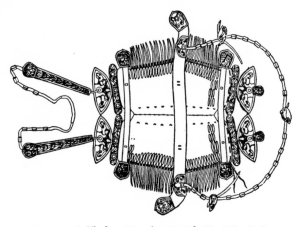

Fig. 37. Saddle from Mound 5, Pazirik. V—IV c. B.C.

with leather covers ornamented with stitching, whilst the wooden frames were bound with red or yellow wool. The cushions were covered with a veritable labyrinth of patterns executed in either felt or leather which was either in appliqué, or encrusted like mosaics, or embossed. Indeed, at times the leather-work came very near to sculpture, so deep was its relief; this relief was given additional height by the addition of leather cut-outs.

Although the Pazirik saddles are the oldest in existence, there is nothing rough or unfinished about them, nor do the elaborate decorations, many of which are in gold, render them unfit for ordinary use. Rudenko strongly disagrees with the suggestion that they may have been intended as show-pieces, for use only at burials, in much the same way that in England in the Middle Ages sham helms were carried at the funerals of knights. All the Pazirik saddles were meant to stand up to hard and regular use; indeed, some show definite signs of consider-able wear and tear. It is perhaps a little difficult today to realize that the nomads never thought of gold as a fragile material, but selected it for a great many objects which they put to constant use. They frequently chose it for covering such resistant basic materials as copper, bronze, iron and wood, and it would never have occurred to them that the presence of gold on a saddle might render it unfit for hard wear.

The marvellously inventive designs which appear on the saddles seldom bear any relation to the elaborate patterns adorning the bridles, yet both are linked by a similar profusion of decorations. The breastbands, which seem to have had a purely ornamental purpose, are perhaps the most spectacular items in the outfits. The motifs which appear on them evolve from a central design which often consists of a bird and a griffin locked in combat, the bird with its wings extended, its feathers veritably sculptured in the thick leather. A griffin with an eagle's beak also frequently appears. So too do stags, goats, leopards and lions, represented either at rest or locked in fight, as well as other contorted, twisted, vibrant animal shapes. The saddle and bridle straps were often decorated either with open-work patterns or silhouettes assuming either geometric forms or taking the shape of mountain goats, cats, leopards, swans, and *Fig. 36* in one instance even of human faces with beards similar in shape to the fake one provided for the Mongoloid chieftain buried at Pazirik. Stags were perhaps the favourite animal motif, but spirals, palmettes, roundels and other floral shapes were the most popular of the purely non-representational patterns. The saddles were often finished off with a decorative binding to the pommel, made of metal, bone, wood or leather. In addition there was an edging of appliqué felt enhanced by ornamental stitching, but sometimes a strand of woollen tassels mounted into wooden terminals was used instead. Occasionally indeed, pieces of gilt wood or bone were carved to represent tassels. The tail straps were worked in surprisingly high relief, the designs chosen for them for the most part consisting of wolves and hares. The saddle cushions, though sufficiently ornate in themselves, were often covered with cases made of either black, white, dark blue or red felt, edged with leather and held in place by narrow leather straps.

Finally, the people of Pazirik added a saddle-cloth to the outfit. The cloths were very large, measuring from twenty-four inches to six feet in length. They were usually made of felt and edged with woollen tassels fitted into wooden terminals. The part of the cloth which was concealed by the saddle was left undecorated, but the remainder was heavily trimmed with appliqué work. The cloth was kept in position by the saddle girth which passed through slots specially made for it. One of the cloths is of particular interest. It was made of a deep cherry-red felt of extreme fineness with strips of woven material mounted on it. Rudenko thinks that the felt was an imported one and he assigns the woven strip to a Persian workshop. One strip displays a geometric pattern formed by tiny columns set in squares; another shows two pairs of women standing on either side of an altar, the entire scene being enclosed in a dog-tooth border; the third displays a row of ominous-looking lions. Another saddle-cloth was made of an exquisite Chinese silk of the shantung type embroidered in many colours with delicate floral motifs and figures of birds. It was edged with blue felt, which was in its turn bordered with a band of red felt adorned with triangular leather appliqués, covered alternately with lead and gold foil. The rest of the cloths were made of local stuffs

Plate 14

Fig. 38

Fig. 39

and decorated with spirited and forceful designs entirely Scythian in style.

Whips appear to have been in general use. At Pazirik many were made of leather with the handles carved in the shape either of horses' heads or else fashioned into an animal's body. In Scythia the whips were usually devoid of carved decorations, but spirals of gold or encrustations of precious materials or gold were added instead.

Both in Scythia and at Pazirik the carts were fitted with a

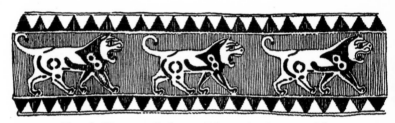

Fig. 38. Woven textile from a Vth-c. B.C. Persian workshop found in Mound 5, Pazirik. Each lion measures 1½ in. long.

central pole some ten feet long with special bow-shaped attachments or cross-pieces measuring six feet or so fixed to it at right angles. The horses were yoked to these cross-pieces in pairs by means of straps. Four horses was the usual number used for pulling the carts, but in southern Russia six often figured at important burials, and at times the number even rose to eight. The driver controlled them from a wooden platform erected at the front of the cart.

Plates 5, 6

In Scythia, but not it would seem at Pazirik, metal standards formed part of a nomad's accoutrements. All those which have been discovered have wooden sockets at their base for fitting on to wooden poles. They have generally been found in groups of four, and Minns supposed that they were attached to the owner's cart, but Smirnov thought that they were fixed to the covered waggons in which the women and children travelled.[2]

The majority display real or mystical animals of heraldic mien, but sometimes birds holding bells in their beaks appear instead.

Fig. 17
DOMESTIC
UTENSILS

As characteristic of the Scythians as their very distinctive horse-trappings are the bronze cauldrons in which they cooked their meat. They have been found in every Scythian burial of any size, and they retained their original shape throughout the entire steppe during the whole of the Scythian age. Most cauldrons other than the Scythian are generally supported by tripod legs which serve to maintain them above the fire. They also have a central hoop handle by which they can be carried and suspended above the flames. But Scythian cauldrons rest on a solid base resembling a truncated cone, and are themselves

Fig. 18

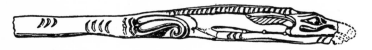

*Fig. 39. Whip handle from Mound 4, Pazirik. V—IV c. B.C.
About 9 in. long.*

virtually hemispherical. Instead of a hoop handle slung from one side to the other, their rims are fitted with two projecting handles which often assume the shape of animals. The Cher-tomlyk cauldron is unusual in having as many as six of these handles. The cauldrons are mostly made out of cast bronze, and they vary in size from quite small examples to those which are over three feet in height and seventy-five pounds in weight. In contrast to almost every other Scythian object, these cauld-rons are seldom decorated, but when their lovely contours are broken by a pattern this is generally confined to a band of stylized arrow-shafts or to some equally restrained geometric composition. The more strongly hellenized Scyths tended to favour somewhat more decoration, but even then it always remained moderate and of a non-representational character. The plainness of the cauldrons was almost certainly dictated by practical considerations, since the smoke from the fires built round the base of the pots would obscure their decoration and render cleaning difficult. The Scythians were not lacking in common sense and, like most traders, they were a thrifty people. Their outlook was typified by their king Arianthus when he organized a census of his people by ordering each man in his kingdom to bring him a bronze arrow-head. Once they had all been counted he arranged for the arrow-heads to be melted down and recast into a great cauldron.

Rostovtzeff[3] identifies a series of vases bearing scenes which are connected with the Great Goddess as sacred vessels. Such

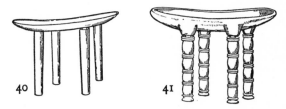

Fig. 40. Table from Mound 4, Pazirik. V c. B.C.
About 1 ft. 4 in. high.

Fig. 41. Table from Mound 3, Pazirik. V c. B.C.
About 1 ft. 4 in. high.

vases come from most Scythian burials irrespective of their locality. These scenes appear most often on rhytons and small-ish, rounded vessels, which Rostovtzeff thinks were reserved exclusively for use at religious ceremonies.

Many of the more valuable drinking vessels which have been found in Scythian graves are of Greek workmanship, but cups that are essentially Scythian also exist. They are characterized by a flattish base and tall, looped handles which probably inspired the shape of Russian wine-tasters of late medieval date. Most nomadic families owned a drinking horn. The kumis jug, another purely Scythian shape, was also a house-hold essential. The finest of these is the Chertomlyk vase. It

Figs. 13, 14

has four spouts ending in animal heads. Three of these have sieves fitted in them, and a fourth sieve is fixed in the vessel's neck. At Pazirik tall pottery jugs were used for storing kumis and not metal ones. They were made locally, in much the same way that the Scythians made the pottery which they needed for everyday use, though they turned to the Greeks for the red-figure ware which they employed at special festivities. From Pazirik we learn that many of the home-made pots were rounded at the base and wooden hoops were used there to maintain them in position. Bowls and flagons, whether of

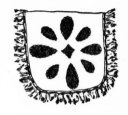

Fig. 42.
Cushion-cover in leather appliqué work from Mound 2, Pazirik. V c. B.C.

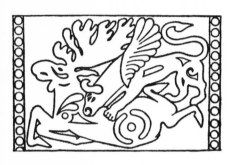

Fig. 43.
Appliqué design from a leather sheet. Mound 2, Pazirik. V c. B.C.

pottery or leather, with similar rounded bases were likewise supported by such hoops, and occasionally stone vessels of the same shape were provided with similar stands.

Plate 15

The Scythians used bone funnels, ladles, colanders, sieves and spoons of many different sizes. They made lamps out of stones, cutting them into small, trough-like rectangles with a tiny leg at each corner as a support.

The Pazirik furniture included square, wooden blocks which could be used either as stools or perhaps even as head-rests. In contrast, their tables were elaborate affairs and surprisingly ingenious. They were low, round or oval in shape and mounted either on turned legs of a startlingly Victorian character, or on legs carved to resemble animals standing upright on their hind legs. The tops were slightly hollowed and

FURNITURE

Figs. 40, 41

137

had bevelled edges. They were detachable and could either be used as trays or else fitted on to the tops of the legs to form tables.

Fig. 42

Mattresses and cushions of various shapes and sizes were stuffed with stag-hair and decorated with the characteristic appliqué work. A hemp-smoking outfit was essential to every nomad, and at Pazirik women as well as men were provided

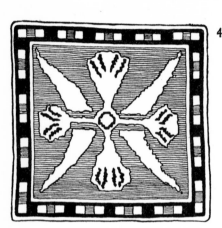

44

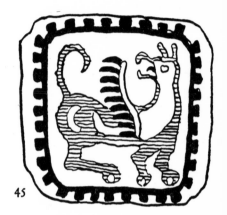

45

Fig. 44. *Star-shaped pattern on pile carpet from Mound 5, Pazirik. V—IV c. B.C.*

Fig. 45. *Griffin on pile carpet from Mound 5, Pazirik. V—IV c. B.C. About 2¼ x 2½ in.*

with a set of their own. At Pazirik some of the cauldrons used by the smokers followed the usual Scythian shape, but sometimes an enlarged version of the little square oil lamps was used instead. Very occasionally round cauldrons with tripod legs and a hoop handle were preferred to the traditional model, for these could be suspended above the fire from the centre of the smokers' tent poles. The tents were often covered with a leather sheet, but sometimes felt ones were substituted instead. In either case, the sheets were left plain, though one of the smokers had

Fig. 43

used a sheet decorated with a row of leopards attacking stags.

That numerous articles of fur were found at Pazirik is not in itself surprising, but it is astonishing to find how skilled the nomads were, even at this early date, at dyeing their furs and working the skins into intricate designs of real quality and merit. Sheep, goat and pony skins were in general use, but leopard fur, skunk, wild cat, squirrel, sable and ermine were regularly

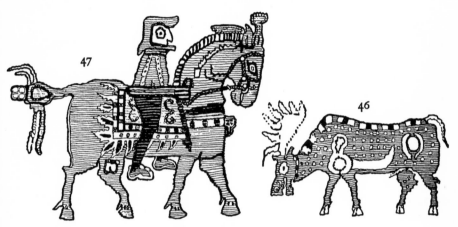

Fig. 46. Elk from pile carpet found in Mound 5, Pazirik. V—IV c. B.C. About 6 x 4 in.

Fig. 47. Rider from pile carpet from Mound 5, Pazirik. V—IV c. B.C. About 9½ x 6½ in.

employed for the better garments, and bags, satchels and pouches were also often made of these furs. Many of the latter were provided with pockets and all had efficient ways of fastening. They were used for carrying cosmetics and mirrors.

Felt was usually chosen for sheets and blankets, but fur and leather were often used. Indeed, the Pazirik people excelled at producing felts of many grades and qualities. They were able also to turn sheep wool into cord and thread, and they knew how to weave, though they do not appear to have been able to produce patterned fabrics. They invariably dyed their thread red and for varying the appearance of their textiles they relied on altering the set of their looms. They appreciated fine textiles, and those which they acquired from their neighbours were of excellent quality. The most interesting of the imports include several Chinese silks of great elegance and the woven strips of Persian material mounted on the red felt saddle-cloth. These strips are dated to the fifth century B.C. Most remarkable of all,

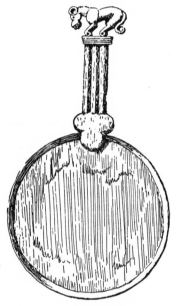

Fig. 48.
Bronze mirror from Romny, south
Russia. Probably of Olbian make.
12 in. long.

however, was the finding in Mound 5 of a Persian pile carpet of very much the same date.

CARPETS   The ancient Greeks had the greatest admiration for carpets of Babylonian and Achæmenid workmanship. Already in their day such rugs were exceedingly valuable and difficult to come by. They often referred to the pile carpets of Sardis,[4] and it may have been rugs of this type that are depicted on the sculptured slabs from Nineveh. These carvings are the earliest pictorial records of rugs to survive to our day, but no carpets nearly as old as the wool-pile rug of the fifth century B.C. discovered at Pazirik were known to the world before the frozen tombs of the Altai disclosed it to our wondering eyes.

The Pazirik carpet scarcely differs at all from the earliest Persian rugs which are still in existence, for although its design is more archaic and its patterns less stylized, the method followed in its making is well-nigh identical to that used until quite recent times throughout the Near East. The carpet measures one metre eighty centimetres by two metres. The central portion is filled with elaborately shaped stars disposed in rows. This section is surrounded by five bands of slightly varying widths. The first of these contains a griffin motif, the next a row of elks walking in single file from right to left, whilst the most interesting strip presents a file of horsemen, their mounts caparisoned in the same style as those appearing on Assyrian sculptures, advancing singly in a stately procession coming from the opposite direction to that taken by the swiftly moving elks. The colours are soft and mellow; the ground a deep red, with other shades of red and a number of pale blues, greens and yellows predominating. The knots number 3,600 to ten square centimetres. Rudenko5 has established that a skilled carpet-maker can tie two thousand knots a day. Since the Pazirik rug contains at least 1,250,000 knots he concludes that it must have taken at least a year and a half to make. He dates it to the fifth century partly on archæological evidence, partly on stylistic grounds, for he considers that the knotting of the horses' tails, their raised forelocks, clipped manes, arched necks, pile saddle-cloths and wide breast-bands are Assyrian features which are closely paralleled in Achæmenid gems of the fifth to the fourth centuries B.C.

Mirrors were an essential in every Scythian household and it seems probable that the important members of the family each possessed a reflector of their own. In southern Russia, alongside the rather small Scythian mirrors with a loop or knob

Fig. 44

Fig. 45
Fig. 46
Fig. 47

MIRRORS

in the centre of the back which rapidly developed into an animal shape, Greek mirrors of the archaic period are frequently found. Some are of Greek workmanship, others are Scythian copies of the Greek, which, with their inveterate love of orna, mentation, and especially their love of zoomorphic forms, their craftsmen covered with decoration. In 1948 the remains of a number of metal workshops were discovered on the site of Olbia with evidence showing that, throughout the sixth and fifth centuries B.C., various objects, more particularly mirrors

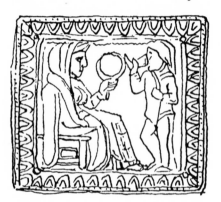

Fig. 49.
Gold costume plaque from
Kul Oba. IV c. B.C.
Perhaps a representation of
the Great Goddess.

and pottery, were made there for selling in Scythia.[6] The earlier mirrors had plain handles with animal terminals, leopards, stags, goats' heads and stylized birds forming the favourite motifs. Scythian mirrors of this date had no handles, and the Olbian ones were exported, together with some cruci, form metal plaques, throughout Scythia, as far afield as Kiev, Hungary and the Urals. In the Altai, as might well be expected, the imported mirrors came from China, the earliest of those found at Pazirik dating from the fifth and fourth centuries B.C.

Mirrors probably served a dual purpose, for although it is evident that the nomads took enough pride in their personal appearance to justify the inclusion of such objects in their graves, it is very probable that, in accordance with primitive

Fig. 48

Fig. 50

belief, mirrors were also considered a helpful accessory in warding off the evil spirits which, as they believed, were ever on the alert to take advantage of mankind. A mirror may also have been regarded as an attribute of the Great Goddess, for a

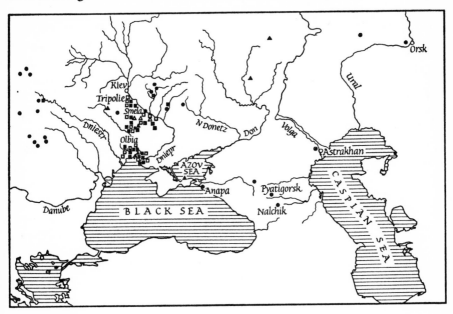

Fig. 50. Map showing extent of Olbian metal-work exports.

small gold plaque from Kul Oba displays a seated female figure which bears a strong likeness to the Pazirik representa-tions of this deity. On the Kul Oba plaque she holds a mirror in her left hand whilst a person stands before her drinking from what may well be a sacred rhyton. At Pazirik, mirrors had very elaborate handles. One of the loveliest had a leather handle and was kept in a most attractive leopard-skin bag decorated with a gold roundel. This mirror probably belonged to the man buried in the grave, for his wife was provided with an exquisite silver mirror mounted on an ox horn. She also owned the only

Fig. 49

stringed instrument found at Pazirik. The other graves contained drums only; these served both to provide music and
to frighten evil spirits away, but her instrument resembled a
lute, whilst one found at Baṣadar foreshadowed the harp.

Bone combs were found at Pazirik, at Neapolis and at a
number of other sites. They were decorated with simple geometric patterns and some had holes cut in the top to allow them
to be tied to the owner's belt. Metal pins and needles were also
found there and they appear regularly and in large numbers in
Scythia proper.

JEWELLERY The Scythians had a veritable passion for adornment,
delighting in decorating themselves no less than their horses and
belongings. Their love of jewellery expressed itself at every turn.
The most magnificent pieces naturally come from the royal
tombs, where the skeletons were invariably bedecked with
golden diadems, head-dresses, necklaces, belts, bracelets, ear-
and finger-rings, torques, pendants, amulets, beads, buttons,
buckles and paste lockets, but even the less important burials
provide an abundance of jewellery and precious materials.
Thus, the skull of the man buried at Sinjavka was decorated
with gold plaques of recumbent stags; at Kelermes either a
barbaric love of jewellery or the primitive dread lest a dead
person's soul should escape from the openings provided by his
nostrils, eye-sockets and ear-holes induced the mourners to fill
the two former with a fine paste inset with precious stones, and
the ears with the type of cloisonné enamelling which is of early
Persian origin. Gold trinkets often smother the bones of the
Plate 16 buried. The majority consist of the small embossed plaques
which they used to trim their clothes with; many of these display
geometric and floral motifs, stylized rosettes and palmettes
being among the most popular of the abstract forms. Animal
representations are even more numerous, and occasionally a
genre scene appears. The latter are of particular interest for they
help to throw light on the Scythian way of life, our only

pictorial records of a musician,[7] or of wrestlers locked in combat[8] coming from such sources. The plaques vary in shape and size, roundels, strips and buttons being very common. Long narrow bands are somewhat rarer, having been used only as head-dress decorations. These head-dresses in their turn vary in form from golden and jewelled diadems, open-work circlets as much as four inches high, or gold skull-caps mounted on leather or red felt, to carved wooden crowns or sculptured leather castles attached, as at Pazirik, to the summit of felt hoods. In the poorer tombs similar objects are for the most part made of bronze or iron rather than of gold, yet even then the same love of finery is expressed with as much skill and delicacy as in the more opulent materials.

Gold frontlets, generally of Greek workmanship, are often found in southern Russia, where bracelets and torques were worn by men and women alike. Indeed, a number of these bracelets deserve to be included with the finest jewellery of the ancient world. In the Caucasus some examples show Achæ-menid influence, but in all of them the Scythians' personal tastes and interests are clearly reflected. The gold plaited chains and necklaces are no less beautiful than the more massive types of jewellery. At Pazirik, primitive neckbands of wood carved with free standing figures of stags and griffins covered in gold-foil and mounted on a bronze hoop resemble in style the no less barbaric and considerably later circlet from Novocherkask, certain details of which in their turn recall the somewhat earlier griffins from the Oxus treasure. Ear-rings are found on most of the bodies; the men wore only one whilst women had two. Finger-rings were universal, and several are often discovered on each finger of both hands. Amulets were very popular, varying from the animal tooth with magical powers and stones of unusual colours and shapes to Assyrian cylindrical seals. At Pazirik silver figurines of horses were worn attached to a belt. Shells and beads were scarcer in the Altai than they were

Plate 20

Plates 17, 18

Plate 21

Fig. 51

amongst the poorer nomads of southern Russia. They are generally found there in quite small graves in conjunction with bronze bracelets, cowrie shells or amulets of rock-crystal, cornelian, amber, bone or paste, each of which sometimes appears in a gold or silver setting.

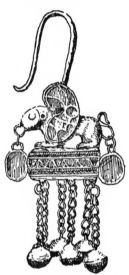

Fig. 51. Gold ear-ring of Graeco-Scythian workmanship from Ryzanovka, Kiev district. Prior to III c. B.C. 2 in. long.

SOURCES

Numbers in parentheses refer to the Bibliography on p. 201.

1 Arendt (52), pp. 206–7.
2 Minns (18), p. 78.
3 Rostovtzeff (27), p. 106, Pl. XXIII.
4 Xenophon (38), V, 5, 7, VIII, 8, 15 and 16.
5 Rudenko (92), pp. 355–6.
6 Bondan (75), p. 58.
7 Minns (18), plaque from belt found at Axjutintsy, fig. 75 *bis*.
8 Rostovtzeff (27), plaque from the lower Dniepr, fourth to third century B.C., Pl. 23, 6.

CHAPTER V

The Art of the Scythian World

WITH THE EXCEPTION of the Pazirik felt hangings, some of which are monumental in character, the art of the nomads working in the Scythian idiom was small in size and essentially decorative in intention, yet practically every object which can be associated with any unit in this group of people possesses many of the attributes essential to a real work of art. Clarity of conception, purity of form, co-ordination of rhythm and balance, and, not least, an understanding and respect for the material employed were triumphantly blended by the Eurasian nomads to produce a distinctive style. The scale on which they worked may have been restricted, the peep-hole through which they gazed on the world may have been limited in size, yet—within these self-imposed boundaries—the outlook was broad, the eye saw with singular clarity and penetration, the mind synthesized with keen lucidity, and the hand gave form to the image which had been thus created with unerring and effortless skill.

The life of these pastoral communities was of necessity so closely bound up with the animals on which their economy was based that the tribesmen developed an acute awareness of the beast world and a far more profound understanding of it than many of us can today realize. This knowledge and the interest which they took in it formed their artistic outlook, leading them to evolve an art which is mainly concerned with animal forms. The state of development which they had themselves reached did not allow of the production of objects whose sole purpose was to give delight. So detached a concept cannot appeal to a primitive people, and indeed most of the great civilizations of the past produced their finest works for reasons other than a purely æsthetic one. The nomads had little reason to create objects in honour of gods or men, but they had an instinct for beauty and the wish to surround themselves with the animal forms in which they had come to delight. These forms had to lend themselves to decorative treatment, for the nomad does not like an art which is liable to stimulate his imagination. Too many dread sounds break the stillness of nights spent in the open steppe, too many queer mirages appear to mislead a tribesman seeking a difficult track, too many weird fancies take possession of him in the lonely hours of his life for him to desire the provocative in art. In a nomadic community, imagination tends to take a sinister road, whereas memory frequently chooses self-deception for a companion and can often gloss over the fearful and unpleasant, to dwell instead on happy and encouraging thoughts.

In a pastoral community the most pleasant memories are generally associated with the chase. The excitement of seeking out the quarry, the thrill on first sighting it—a thrill which is often accompanied by a twinge of admiration for the victim— the successful outcome of the hunt, all this provides material for a glorious tale to be recounted to an admiring audience at the close of day. The more exciting details continue to remain fresh in the mind long after the narrative has lost much of its savour. Most vividly enduring are the dramatic incidents, the mental picture of the moment when the tracked creature, first sensing the approaching danger, stops to sniff the air with distended nostrils, then bounds away in a wild gallop in search of safety, till, at last, struck by the death-inflicting arrow, it collapses to the ground, not in an ugly heap as does a dying man, but with elegance and resignation.

Like some of the prehistoric paintings of northern Spain and south-western France, those which Lamaev discovered in 1940 in the almost inaccessible gorge of Zarautsay in Uzbekistan depict hunting scenes.[1] Paintings of this type were essentially magical in intention and their artistic merits are thus largely

fortuitous. But in neolithic Siberia, that is to say during the
third millennium, life-size figures of animals were often carved in
bone or wood to serve as decoys. Eding[2] found some shaped as
ducks whilst excavating in the Gorbunovski Bog in the
Nijnetagil county in the district of Sverdlovsk in Siberia. These
decoys were at first completely naturalistic in style, but with the
centuries the naturalism of such works tended to give way to a
certain stylization. As the refinement in style became more
marked, so did the symbolism which had been originally
associated with certain beasts and scenes tend to be forgotten.
Yet the designs which had lost some of their religious meaning
continued to persist as decorations, surviving partly through
force of habit, partly because they continued to please. An
æsthetic element was thus introduced to the field of pictorial
representation, and this in its turn resulted in the development
of a more complex style. With the Scythians it became essential
for animal designs, irrespective of their religious significance, to
please the eye by confronting it with a thoroughly convincing
rendering of its subject and to satisfy memory by producing a
synthesis of the creature's fundamental characteristics as seen at
various moments of its existence. The nomads therefore tried to
combine in a single rendering all the salient points of the animal
they were delineating, showing it simultaneously in motion,
with its front legs still pounding the air, and at rest, with the
back legs in a recumbent posture. A motion picture would
have fulfilled the Scythians' requirements; even a strip cartoon
would have delighted them. Indeed, they came nearer to inventing the latter than did the Sumerians with their cylinder
seals, though these may well have served as a source of Scythian
inspiration.

The nomads achieved considerable success in the difficult task
of showing in a single image the various and often incompatible
poses assumed by a single animal in the course of its life. The
extended outline of a swiftly moving creature—the flying gallop

as it has been called—is the supreme expression of their art, even though the creature's head and forelegs may be shown frontally, whereas the hind-quarters may convolute in the opposite direction so as to recall the collapse of a stricken beast. It is difficult to feel that figures of this sort—perhaps the nearest to pure abstraction ever achieved by representational art—had any deeply religious meaning attached to them. The images are too redolent of life, too analytical and dispassionate, the grouping of the animals is too haphazard, the repertory of beasts too wide and the poses too varied for this to be likely. Tradition may well have dictated the motifs, for Scythian art followed definite forms and conventions, but religion cannot have had any influence.

The nomads reacted to their surroundings with an unusually acute sensitivity, and just as the Eurasian plain vibrated with life, so, in the highly impressionistic and symbolic language of their art, did they attempt to express this universal vitality by means of ingeniously contrived zoomorphic junctures. An *Fig. 52* extremity of one animal thus developed into an attribute of another. Frankfort[3] suggested that the Scythians might have acquired the idea from the Lurs, but if so the Lurs must themselves have learnt it from the Hittites, who delighted in turning the tail of one animal into the head of another. The habit of filling a vacant space by permitting part of one creature to turn into the distinguishing feature of another was ascribed by Minns to a fear or dislike of the void, but it seems more in keeping with their imagery to interpret it as an intuitive response to the diversity and versatility of nature. The idea of experimenting in this way may have reached the Scythians direct from the Hittites, for the princely burials which Kuftin excavated at Trialeti,[4] a hundred miles or so from Tiflis, produced quantities of gold and silver objects, many of which show definite signs of Hittite origin. Other finds of the same type, almost as rich, were found by Pietrovsky[5] at Kirov Han in Armenia. They must in consequence have been imported direct from Asia Minor.

Most of the animals which appear in Scythian art played an important part in the arts of the civilizations which flourished in Egypt and the Ancient Orient from the fourth millennium onwards. Though some forms originated in one area, some in another, they spread throughout the civilized world of the time and became familiar all over it. Animals of every sort, whether real or imaginary, were thus depicted by artists of every race, though in the style proper to each region. In the Middle East the representations remained strongly naturalistic till well into the Sumerian age, when heraldic compositions began to appear. Among the most popular of the new motifs was a group of three figures, consisting either of a human being, a tree, or an animal flanked by heraldic beasts. The central figure first represented the god Gilgamesh and the beasts the power of darkness with which he was in eternal strife, but the Scythians transformed him into the Great Goddess and the animals into her attendants. Hunting scenes came into prominence in central Asia at much the same date. Fabulous beasts made their entry gradually, but from about 3000 B.C. their curious shapes figure flamboyantly in the art of Mesopotamia. In the second millennium fierce lions with scowling faces came to guard the entrances to the citadels, palaces and temples of the Hittite empire. Creatures of every sort kept a constant watch on the monuments erected by the Assyrians, and at the magnificent palace of Persepolis winged lions attacking oxen proclaimed the importance of strength from the political as well as the religious point of view. On the south-eastern fringe of Eurasia griffins of both the lion- and the eagle-headed varieties kept constant, if less spectacular guard over the valuable gold deposits of Siberia and Tibet.

Fig. 16

By this time northern Syria, Upper Mesopotamia, most of Anatolia, the whole of the Armeno-Caucasian area and much of Persia formed a single cultural unit. Attempts to trace the source of the animal style in Scythian art have proved unrewarding, for the tracks are numerous and lead in many directions. Thus Rostovtzeff looked to central Asia for the origins of the style, Tallgren to Russian Turkestan, Borovka to northern Siberia, Schmidt to the Ancient Orient and Ebert to Ionia and the coast of the Black Sea. In actual fact Scythian art is a compound of elements pertaining to all these regions built round a distinct core of its own.

In the Caucasus an animal art in a style of its own had evolved long before the Scythians appeared in the area. The royal tombs at Maikop date from the third millennium, but it is there that gold plaques first appear as trimmings for clothes. Its votive bronze statuettes of bulls and stags are in a style which to some extent affected the earliest examples of animal art so far discovered in Anatolia, in the pre-Hittite works from Alaça Hüyük. Frankfort[6] drew attention to their influence on the copper statuettes of bulls found there, and Vieyra[7] suggests that these Maikop characteristics may have been brought to the region by people who migrated to Anatolia from the Caucasus. Piggott[8] is no less conscious of the link. But Maikop was not an isolated achievement. The last thirty years have produced a good deal of evidence to show that metal-workers were established at many points in the Caucasus from the early bronze age onwards. Kuftin found clear proof of this both at Trialeti and at Kirov Han, and Gobedjishvili uncovered the remains of important metal workings, as well as workshops containing moulds and castings dating from the second millennium B.C., close to the village of Gebi on the upper Riom river in the Caucasus.[9] The Maikop objects must have been produced by a similar group of metal-workers, and in each case the craftsmanship is so accomplished and the style so evolved that it is evident that these works must have had a long line of forebears behind them. Yet their ancestors defy identification, though all contributed in forming the art of the Eurasian nomads.

Scythian metal-work also shows distinct traces of having

Fig. 53

evolved from wood or bone carving, and some scholars have therefore sought for its origin north of the Eurasian plain, among the Eskimo carvers from the shores of the White Sea and the Sea of Bering.[10] In that case the first tentative carvings of the northerners must have undergone a long process of evolution in Siberia and the Caucasus before they developed into the stylized and elaborate forms preserved in the Scythian horses' bits and cheek-pieces, where this native style survives in its purest form.

The impact of the Middle East resulted in the inclusion of a number of new animal scenes in Caucasian art. After the eighth century B.C., by which time the Assyrians had subdued the Syrians and Phœnicians, the oriental influence became more marked. Then the Scythian advance across Asia brought the Caucasian area into touch with Egypt and statuettes of the god Bes penetrated to western Siberia,[11] and to Kiev and its neighbourhood, whilst the lotus appeared at Pazirik.[12]

Of all the many elements which made themselves felt in Scythian art the strongest was perhaps the Ionian. It penetrated to Eurasia from several directions. In the first instance it reached the nomads from Persia, where Ionian workmen were employed on building Darius' great palace at Susa,[13] but it was also brought direct from Ionia by the merchants trading with the towns on the eastern shores of the Black Sea and it was in addition disseminated throughout southern Russia by the Greek artists working at Panticapaeum and at other points in the northern Pontus. The Scythians delighted in the elegance of Ionian art, but they were equally alive to the beauty and opulence of Persian art, savouring its grandeur and dignity.

The earliest known Scythian tombs are contemporary in date with the Scythians' military successes in the Middle East and in consequence the majority are situated in the eastern extremity of the European section of the plain. Close to them in date are some of the south Russian mounds. Three of the earliest burials, those of Kostromskaya Stanitza, Kelermes in the Kuban, the Melgunov barrow in southern Russia, and a hoard discovered fairly recently in Sakiz in Urartu, on the probable site of the Scythians' first capital,[14] are of particular importance. Ghirshman has been able to assign the Sakiz finds to the years 681–668 B.C. on the basis of details of costume, but the burials are more difficult to place. The Melgunov barrows are generally accepted as belonging to the second half of the sixth century B.C., but there is disagreement over the dating of the Kelermes and Kostromskaya burials. Thus Rostovtzeff ascribed them to the sixth century, whereas Borovka and other Soviet authorities date them to the seventh. Whatever the dating, it is significant that the Scythian style already appears fully developed in all four sites, and the discovery of earlier burials, belonging to the Scythian period of obscurity, must be awaited before the evolution of their art can be traced with any detail.

The objects found in these four sites reflect Persian influence. A sword sheath from Melgunov[15] shows the successful fusion of the native and Assyrian elements, for the sword itself is Persian in shape, and the decorations on the sheath also display strong Assyro-Persian trends. The main design thus consists of a row of Persian-looking winged quadrupeds, alternately human- and lion-headed, advancing with drawn bows. Their wings are, however, essentially Scythian, for instead of being formed of feathers, they consist of fish which maintain themselves in position by clinging with their teeth to the bowmen's shoulders. The latter do not seem to suffer from this very early and unusually savage example of zoomorphic juncture. Another Middle-Eastern element consists in the indication of the muscles on the creatures' legs by dot and comma markings. This detail reappears constantly in the animal art of the ancient world. It is to be seen on many Persian sculptures of early date as well as on the woven strip of material of Persian origin displaying lions found at Pazirik. It appears too at Alaça

Fig. 52

Fig. 38

Hüyük,[16] and it is impossible to determine whether the Scythians adopted the markings from the later Hittites or from the Persians, or to discover where else the markings originated. Another Persian motif decorates the hilt of the same sheath, in this case a representation of an Assyrian altar set between two trees. This again bears some resemblance to the altar shown on the second woven Persian fragment found at Pazirik, but in contrast the side projection to the sheath is adorned with the

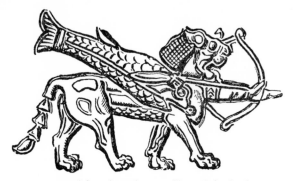

Fig. 52. Detail from the Melgunov gold sword sheath. $1\frac{3}{4}$ x 1 in.

beautifully modelled figure of a recumbent stag, which often serves as the hall-mark of Scythian workmanship.

Persian influence is again reflected in the gold-work from Kelermes. A sword sheath from this burial is well-nigh identical with the Melgunov example. Quite outstanding is the figure of a leopard from the centre of a round shield, having enamel inlay of the Persian type applied to it; a gold diadem and other pieces of jewellery have been found similarly adorned. A symbolic axe was covered with gold decorations primarily Scythian in character. Its handle displays the figures of various recumbent animals disposed in rows, though the projecting end of the axe is rather more Persian in style. By it lay a silver mirror of the finest Ionian workmanship, its decorations consisting of various animals, centaurs and monsters. A dish showing the

Plate 9

Great Goddess was another notable find.

The Kostromskaya barrow is distinguished by some unusual features of construction, but it is primarily noted for the impor-tance of its contents. In it, among other magnificent objects, were found an iron scale hauberk with shoulder scales of copper and, loveliest of all, the gold figure of a recumbent stag, which is one of the glories of Scythian art.

Plate 23

At Sakiz[17] some purely Assyrian pieces of jewellery and plate were found beside some outstanding examples of early Scythian workmanship. The latter include a gold sword sheath decorated with ibex heads and somewhat coarse human heads, a gold plaque with lynx heads alternating with the figures of recumbent ibexes and Scythian-looking stags, and, most exciting of all, a large silver dish, measuring some fourteen inches in diameter. It was entirely covered with decoration, the main patterns being disposed in rows or contained within con-centric bands. One band enclosed a row of crouching creatures facing to the left, whilst another had a row of hares looking in the opposite direction and yet another displayed animal heads likewise facing to the right. The disposition of creatures or people moving in opposite directions recalls the design of the pile carpet found at Pazirik, where the horsemen and stags advance in such a manner. On Mesopotamian seals dating from 3500–3000 B.C. bands of animals are sometimes shown walking in opposite ways.[18] The idea was never carried any further there, nor does it appear in Persian sculpture, but it can be seen in embryo on the famous silver vase from Maikop,[19] where one bull stands with his back to the others, and on a silver mug of much the same date from Trialeti,[20] where the decoration is divided into two horizontal bands. The lower section shows stags walking in single file from right to left whilst, in the upper, a chieftain seated on a throne beside a holy tree flanked by sacrificial animals, watches a procession of twenty-three half-animal, half-human, Hittite-looking creatures

Fig. 53

which approach from the left. The idea reaches full development as a decorative device only in Scythian metal-work; an
early example is the Sakiz dish, a late one the Chertomlyk
cauldron, where the two central goat-shaped handles face in
opposite ways. Rudenko assigns the Pazirik carpet to a Persian

Fig. 18

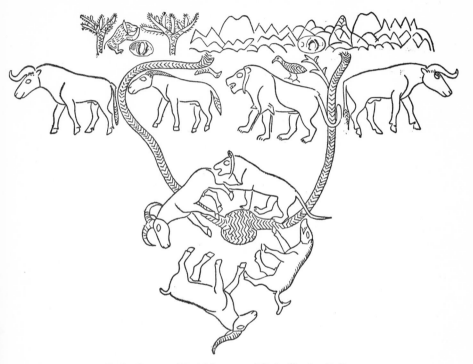

Fig. 53. Design from one of the Maikop vases. Third millennium B.C.

workshop, but since the disposition of its decoration seems more
characteristic of Scythia, it may have been made to the express
order of a Pazirik chieftain. The appearance two centuries
earlier, at Sakiz, of a similar decorative arrangement seems to
suggest that designs consisting of creatures moving in opposite
ways within enclosed bands are of Scythian origin.

Among the decorations on the Sakiz dish are some which resemble creatures found at Kelermes and Melgunov. Thus, with but one notable exception, all the most characteristic motifs of Scythian art are already found in their fully developed form at the four earliest sites which can be associated with the Scythians. The exception consists of scenes showing one or more animals attacking another animal, for the fish-wing of the Melgunov sheath represents a zoomorphic juncture and not a combat scene.

The most characteristic single motif in Scythian art is provided by the stag. Originally an object of worship among Siberian tribesmen, it had probably lost much of its earlier religious significance by Scythian times, but it is more than likely that the belief that stags transported the souls of the dead to the world beyond[21] was still generally current in Eurasia throughout the first millennium. It persisted with the Buriats until quite recently. This probably accounts for the stag's presence on funerary objects, and may help to explain the

Plates 11, 12, *Fig. 29*

antlered horse-masks found at Pazirik, where the mourners may well have hoped to speed the journey of their dead by endowing the horses, through the intermediary of the head-dresses, with the additional swiftness of a stag or a bird. The

Fig. 26

stag motifs decorating the coffin from Mound 2 at Pazirik are portrayed with great realism, and it is perhaps significant that they are shown running, whereas those which appear on objects unconnected with the funeral are often shown at rest, and are so strongly stylized that it is difficult to feel that they were intended for any purpose but that of decoration. The finest gold figures of stags are of relatively early date. The larger ones often formed the centre-pieces of shields and are usually of moulded gold.

Plate 23

The beautiful stag from Kostromskaya Stanitza dates from the seventh or sixth century B.C. It is in a recumbent position, with its legs tucked beneath it so that the underneaths of its hooves are visible. Though triangular in shape, they are not exaggeratedly so, and although the stag is lying, or rather crouching, its head is raised so that its antlers rest along its back. Its neck is extended as though it were moving at speed, like a great glider travelling into the face of the wind, the sensitive, twitching nostril seeming to provide motive power. The eye is round, the expression one of apprehension, the muscles of the neck and body so taut that, although the animal is shown at rest, it gives an impression of rapid, easy motion. This stag is a superb example of a type which recurs with small variations on divers objects of different sizes and dates.

Another important, if not quite so satisfying example comes from Kul Oba in the Crimea. It is to be dated to the middle of the fourth century B.C., and this comparatively late dating is borne out by stylistic considerations, for although the stag itself is beautifully modelled, comparison with the Kostromskaya version reveals something slightly mechanical in the treat- ment of the antlers. In this case the stylization is monotonous, the ear almost unrecognizable, the eye somewhat clumsy and the upturned feet exaggeratedly pointed. These features suggest an urban metal-worker's rather than a nomad's hand. The filling in of the blank spaces on the body with smaller animal forms is again a pseudo-nomadic rather than a purely Scythian device. The Vettersfeld[22] fish, which is almost con- temporary in date, being no earlier than the first decades of the fifth century B.C., is no less splendidly modelled than the Kul Oba stag and is similarly marred by the incongruous insertion on its body of various scenes and animals which, though skil- fully executed, are extraneous to the design. Both objects must have come from the same workshop, and it is tempting to assign them to a Greek from Olbia who had failed to dis- tinguish between a zoomorphic juncture, which serves to complement a design, and this type of filling in, which breaks its unity. The criticism is not applicable to the splendid bronze standard of the sixth century B.C. from Mound 2 at Ulski.

Plate 24

Plate 5

Here the design is so highly stylized that the animal forms which went to its making have lost their identity in the geometry of the pattern, which serves as a frame for the little heraldic stag set in the space left blank to receive it.

Plate 25

A magnificent gold stag from Tapioszentmarton in Hungary shows a greater purity of conception than does the Kul Oba example. It comes closer to the Kostromskaya stag, from which it is clearly descended. The limbs are outlined with delicate granulations, the legs clearly indicated; its feet are carefully shaped, with the hooves still turned upwards. Originally the eye-sockets and ear-holes were filled with enamel, suggesting Persian influence, yet this is probably once again a Greek work, for granulations of this type are not typical of Scythian work-manship. The stag is of comparatively early date, certainly not later than the fifth century or so B.C.

Figures of fish are fairly common, though they are more fre-quent in Siberia than in Scythia. In the Near East fish were invested with religious significance and in the Caucasus they survived in legends, and retained a certain symbolic meaning till well into Christian times. Large figures of fish hewn out of stone, called vishaps, are still to be found on high vantage points in Armenia, where they were probably installed for ritualistic purposes at a time when they personified the weather god.[23] In Scythian art they are characteristic of the archaic period. At Pazirik they appear quite frequently, and one was Fig. 28 included in the designs tattooed on the Mongoloid chieftain's leg.

The use of coloured inlay was a device which had been resorted to as far back as the days of Ur's magnificence, but nowhere in the ancient world was it more splendidly or lavishly applied than in Achæmenid Persia.[24] The Scythians must have learnt this delicate technique from Persia, for objects of but slightly earlier date from Siberia are generally still adorned with inset stones rather than with enamel. The Scythian fondness for inlay was especially marked during the earlier years of their ascendancy and there is no indication that the kindred tribes ever used this difficult and expensive form of decoration. A beautiful, early example of inlay is afforded by the gold leopard found at Kelermes which is modelled with the same subtle forcefulness as the virtually contemporary stag from Kostromskaya. A liking for inlay was not confined to the Kuban. From Altin Oba in the Crimea, comes an exquisite figurine of sixth to fifth century date of a lioness in cast bronze. It is covered with gold foil, and the central portion of its body is formed of tiny, vertical gold partitions filled with inlay. Here again, as in the Kelermes leopard, the creature's toes and cheeks are marked by chasing.

    Single animal figures such as these are the masterpieces of Scythian art, but compositions showing one or more creatures linked in combat are scarcely less characteristic or lovely. The motif, itself of great antiquity, became very popular in Scythia, but nowhere was it expressed with such fervour as in the Altai. An early, essentially Scythian version as opposed to an Altaian one, comes from The Seven Brothers Barrow in the Kuban, where a wooden rhyton of the early fifth century B.C. was decorated with four gold plaques. Each one shows a bird of prey or a carnivorous animal attacking a herbivorous one. On the plaque illustrated here a winged lion is seen attacking a mountain goat; its claws have seared the victim's flank as it takes a bite out of its back, yet the goat sits erect and impassive. Only the agonized expression of its eye gives any indication of the pain it is enduring.

    A splendid gold stag from Zoldhalompuszta in Hungary seems to belong to the same group of designs as The Seven Brothers plaque, for the creature's terrified expression and the impression of imminent flight so sensitively conveyed by its raised leg surely indicate that, in its original state, the stag was shown being pursued by some beast of prey. Once again the

Plate 9

Plate 26

Plate 27

Plate 28

limbs and muscles are powerfully modelled, and notwith-standing the hint at motion, the creature is still shown in a static position. This almost passive attitude links it to the vic-tims on The Seven Brothers' rhyton. Nevertheless, the granula-tions on the stag's legs and tail, the curious scallop-like pattern outlining the base of its neck, and the insertion of a bird's head at the base of the antlers, point to Greek influence. These details link it to the Kul Oba stag and preclude an earlier dating than the fifth century B.C.

Plate 24

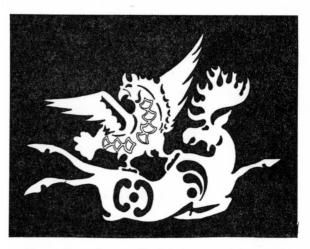

Fig. 54. Design from a saddle-cloth from Mound 1, Pazirik.
V c. B.C. About 12 x 7½ in.

The Pazirik people handled the same motif rather differently from the Scythians. It recurs constantly on their objects, form-ing the main decoration for articles of every type, yet never becoming dull or repetitive. One version, but only one, is static in character, showing two animals of the same species, one a lion-headed griffin and the other an eagle-headed one, which are thus both of equal rank, confronting each other. This is not properly speaking a combat scene; it is either a symbolic

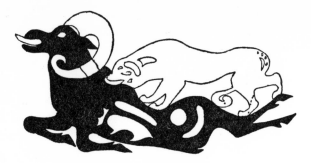

Fig. 55. Design from a saddle from Mound 1 Pazirik, V c. B.C.
15 x 6 in.

composition, the meaning of which is now lost to us, or a
purely decorative design. A semi-static version from a saddle
from Mound 2 at Pazirik is also not exactly a combat scene. By
presenting an eagle or crested griffin triumphantly erect as it
digs its claws into the palpitating body of a conquered stag, it
registers the moment of victory rather than a stage in the fight.

Fig. 54

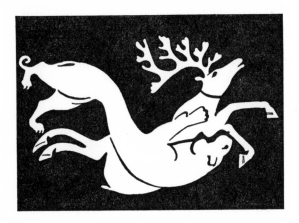

Fig. 56. Design from a saddle-cloth from Mound 1, Pazirik.
V c. B.C. About 18 x 10 in.

Fig. 55

Another saddle-cloth from the same mound records the moment of impact rather than that of achievement. It shows a tiger landing with all four feet on the body of a mountain goat. As the creature collapses under the attack, with its front legs bent beneath its chest, its rump turned outwards and its hind legs uselessly extended, the tiger digs its fangs into the quivering flesh. Although the design is carried out in appliqué felt, leather and gold foil cut-outs, all but the last of which are materials lacking in glamour, an astonishing emotional and rhythmic effect has been achieved, the stylized handling of the animals' bodies preserving their essential anatomical character-istics intact, whilst the rounded lines of the composition justify Hogarth's faith in the beauty of the curved line.

Fig. 56

No less rhythmic is the scene from a saddle-cloth found in Mound 1 at Pazirik showing a tiger pursuing a stag. In this version the tiger has sprung to attack, but has not as yet wounded his prey. Both animals are locked in fight as they hurtle through the air, their bodies intertwined in an altogether impossible manner which nevertheless succeeds admirably in evoking several phases of the fight. Each has its rump turned outward in a way which is wholly contrary to nature, but which is nevertheless thoroughly convincing. The combat

Figs. 57–60

scenes tattooed on the body of the Mongoloid chief from Mound 2 at Pazirik, though equally fantastic, depicting ani-mals completely unreal, with attributes so improbable that veracity retires defeated from the field, seem no less authentic than the scenes involving actual animals. The extraordinarily powerful impression of rapid, almost frenzied motion and force created by these Pazirik designs has seldom been surpassed in drawing. Their popularity persisted in Asia well into this era. A magnificent woollen carpet, quilted and adorned with appliqué work, found beneath the coffin of a first century A.D. Hunnic chieftain buried at Noin Ula in northern Mongolia,

Plate 29

includes in its border the scene of a griffin attacking a stag[25]

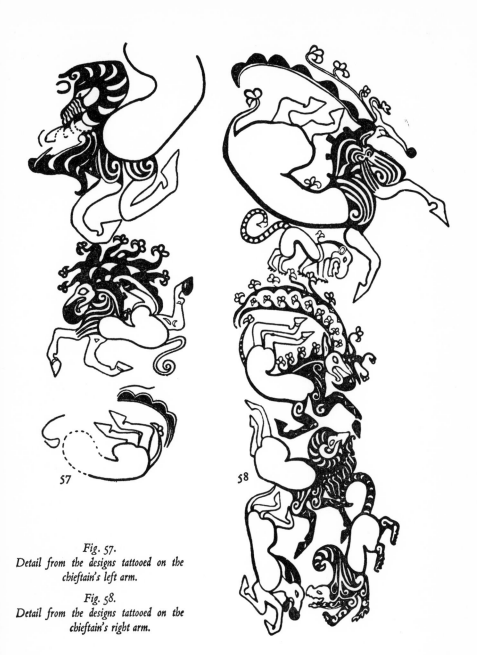

Fig. 57.
Detail from the designs tattooed on the
chieftain's left arm.

Fig. 58.
Detail from the designs tattooed on the
chieftain's right arm.

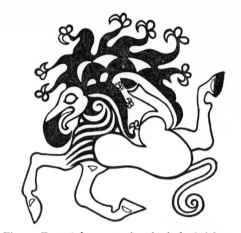

Fig. 59. Fantastic beast tattooed on the chieftain's left arm.

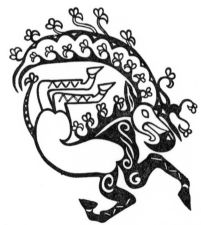

Fig. 60. Fantastic beast tattooed on the chieftain's right arm.

and shows that the mastery persisted throughout many centuries.

A most unusual combat scene of quite exceptional interest decorated a wall-hanging found in Mound 5 at Pazirik. The hanging originally measured a little over a yard in length, with the scene forming a frieze along it. Both the combat scene and

Fig. 61

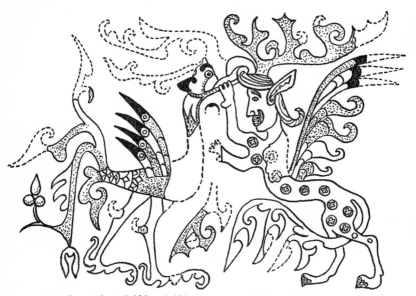

Fig. 61. Antlered, half-lion, half-human creature fighting a fantastic bird from a felt hanging found in Mound 5, Pazirik. V—IV c. B.C.

the border round it were executed in coloured felt appliqués, the combatants appearing on a white ground. The right-hand figure has survived almost intact. Half-man, half-lion, it might well have stepped from the world of the Hittites, but Rudenko links it with the sphinx, even though the face with its black moustache points to Assyria rather than to Egypt or Eurasia. Its pale blue lion-like body is studded with brown rosettes. It stands upright on lion feet which have large claws that provide a parallel to those belonging to one of the creatures tattooed on the dead chieftain's back. Its long tail is elegantly tucked between its legs, to swing out at the level of its chest in a cluster of leaf-like terminals. A wing rises from the centre of its back, its side feathers forming S-shaped squiggles not altogether unlike those used to indicate the antlers belonging to the Kostromskaya stag. Its hands are extended and the newly completed restorations of the fragments[26] show that they are directed at attacking a bird-like figure with a somewhat human face, crowned by either antlers or a large crest. But the most interesting feature is perhaps the magnificent antlers which tower above the head of the first combatant. The scene is assuredly imbued with some deep mystical meaning.

When this figure is considered in conjunction with the in-numerable representations of antlers and horns which appear in the art of the Eurasian nomads it becomes abundantly clear that antlers played a most important part in the religious rituals of a number of vastly different peoples throughout many millennia of the prehistoric age. Salmony[27] has in fact traced their sporadic appearance as a religious emblem as far west as the cave of Les Trois Frères at Montesquieu-Avantès in France, where they are found on a carved and painted figure of a half-human, half-animal creature. The Hunter's Camp at Star Carr in Yorkshire produced several sets of antlers which had quite obviously figured in ritual observances, and antlers had already appeared with much the same purpose in early Hittite art. Nowhere, however, was their symbolic use more wide-spread than in the eastern section of the Eurasian plain. The Scythian word for stag served as the tribe's totemic name,[28] the animal and its antlers are favourite motifs of Scythian art. There it frequently retained much of its original symbolic meaning, but at the same time, the happy-go-lucky nomads, regardless of whether they belonged to a purely Scythian or a kindred tribe, did not hesitate often to subject the once entirely sacred antler pattern to their innate love of artistry. Their passion for decoration was thus responsible for the fine and unusually well-balanced design preserved on a bronze horse frontlet of the fourth century B.C. coming from the Kuban. In this well-thought-out composition the central motif consists of the side view of a stag's head framed in a frontal, symmetrical arrangement of antlers. This main pattern is flanked on one side by the zoo-morphically joined heads of three birds and on the other by a stag's head, set this time at right angles to the central design so that the antlers counterbalance the birds' heads. The result-ing pattern is strikingly decorative and comes very close to abstract art.

Plate 32

   If any real advance is to be made in our understanding of the outlook and beliefs of the Asiatic peoples of the first millennium B.C., the antler problem will have to be solved. It carries the searcher right into China, to the province of the Hunan, where a small group of carved wooden human and animal figures, all of them adorned with antlers, were discovered at Ch'ang-sha, in a group of tombs exposed during building operations. One of these figures—a human head with a protruding tongue is now preserved in the British Museum; all of them have been fully published by Salmony. In trying to establish the signifi-cance of the antler emblem, Salmony[29] came across a reference in the Shan Hai Ching text, parts of which date back to Han times, to creatures having animal bodies and human faces topped with antlers or horns, which may perhaps represent variants of the Pihsieh, a mythical, antlered creature resembling a stag, capable of averting the evil eye, mentioned in a legend from north China. In this connection Salmony reminds his readers that the Buddhists included eleven deer symbols in their earliest legends, that the Tibetans, and until quite recent times the Shamans of Siberia, retained the use of antlers in their ceremonial robes, and that antlers also played some part in the life of Celtic Ireland and medieval England and Scandinavia.

Plate 31

The use of antlers at Ch'ang-sha must assuredly be ascribed to nomadic influence. Salmony recognizes that, in Eurasia, the stag cult was indigenous and dates back into prehistory, and it is thus not without significance that the Chinese his-torians mentioned by Salmony described the inhabitants of the Hunan during the latter half of the first millennium B.C. as 'semi-Barbaric' and affirmed that they differed radically from the people in the rest of China. No antler-crowned figures have as yet been found anywhere else in China excepting the Hunan, and all those which have so far been discovered date from the fourth to the third centuries B.C., the very period when the Asiatic, or at any rate the Altaian nomads were at the height of their prosperity. The antlers on one of the Ch'ang-sha figures, that of a double-headed animal now in the Cox collection at Washington, like so many objects found at Pazirik and Katanda, were made of bark, and this seems to confirm that the objects were produced under nomadic influence and that the clue to the antler problem is to be sought in Siberia.

The nomads decorated their harness with both animal and geometric designs. Every variety of animal appears on them, though stags and eagles are perhaps most numerous. Antler designs, geometric and floral motifs, birds' heads surmounted with cocks' combs, griffins with features of a suslik appear in low and high relief, in silhouette or cut-out, and occasionally in the round. Feline creatures are to be numbered among the most charming works, many a one recalling the opening lines of Pushkin's poem, *Ruslan and Ludmila*, where:

Plate 39

> A green oak stands on the water brink,
> With a golden chain it is bound.
> A salient cat on each winding link
> Day and night goes round and round;
> When he goes to the right, a song he sings;
> To the left, a tale he brings.

The bone carvings reflect the native style more clearly perhaps than does the metal-work. The heads of a ram from Kelermes and of a fierce beast, probably a wolf, from the Black Mountains of the Orenburg district show how little change was necessary to adapt the technique of carving, whether in bone or wood, to that of working in metal. The Pazirik people were fond of covering their wood carvings with beaten gold or lead foil, but even when working in plain wood, they produced works which are veritable masterpieces of their kind, such as for example the head of a mountain goat or the head of an ibex. Whatever the scale, the figures remain beautifully proportioned, and the less costly material is as skilfully and considerately treated as the most precious, so that objects in bronze are artistically in no way inferior to those in gold, nor are designs made of felt any less satisfactory than those produced in wood. In Persia the skill survived into this century and the figure of an ibex which I once saw, made of dried figs by a Turki nomad camping near Shapur some twenty years ago, must surely stand as the last in a long line of animal forms produced by Asiatic nomads.

Plate 36
Plate 34

Plates 38, 40

In Scythian times figures of stags, ibexes, bulls or some other animal, with their feet gathered together on a knob were made in the round to serve as pole tops or furniture terminals. The form is often associated with the Scythians, but it is of far greater antiquity, having already appeared on Amrathian ivory combs of the fourth millennium.[30] It is curious that although the horse played an all-important part in the daily lives of the nomads, it seldom figures in their art. An early example occurs on the silver vessel from Maikop and horses continue to appear here and there throughout the centuries. They were popular at Kelermes, and figure on the vessels which the Greeks made for the Scythians, and they are found occasionally at Pazirik, where they sometimes appear as amulets.

Plates 57–9

The nomads saw everything as a pattern, and they found it

Figs. 62, 63

no more difficult to turn an animal shape into a geometric form than to transform a pattern into an animal attribute. So, for example, a spirited ram from a saddle-cloth in Mound 1 at Pazirik has the curly ruff round its head made from a pattern which may equally well have been derived from an axe-head as from a beast's horn. The same motif appears in its former character on a horse's tail-sheath from the same mound.

The impact which all these animal forms make on the mind is extremely sharp. The rich variety of the creatures themselves is no less impressive than the diverse aspects in which they appear. Real and imaginary, probable and altogether unlikely beasts jostle and confront each other, intertwine and intermix with such exuberant abandonment and venom that a new, unexpected and unexplored world unfolds before us. As we venture into this strange land, a taut muscle here, a frightened eye beyond, a magnificent antler ahead, all conspire to render the scene familiar and real, reviving a memory carelessly noted during the chase and quickly forgotten in its excitement. Interspersed in the background are solar symbols and geometric patterns disposed with consummate artistry.

Fig. 34

At Pazirik the love of decoration expressed itself at every turn. Arrows, whose lot it was to fly but once through the keen air, were painted with meanders and spirals as elegant as any which appear on objects intended for more frequent use. Straps of every sort were embellished with open-work patterns cut in diamonds, stars, hearts, crosses, rosettes, palmettes, lotus flowers and petal motifs. The saddle-cloths have the quality of splendid carpets. The human form alone plays a very small part in this art. In Scythia the majority of the human figures were produced by Greek artists living close at hand and they never seem to have inspired the Scythians to emulate them. Occasionally, more as a joke and rather in the manner of a Romanesque grotesque, both in Scythia and at Pazirik a face would be carved on some ornament, but the designer's heart was seldom in the work, and at Pazirik, the man carving a face on a wooden tassel was unable to resist the temptation of turning the top of its head into a palmette. Yet the Eurasians could have produced human forms had they wished to do so. This is evident from

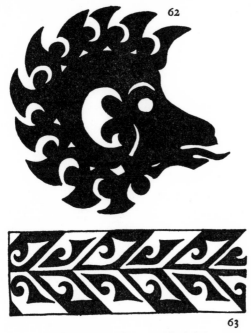

Fig. 62. A ram's head worked in felt on a saddle-cloth from Mound 1, Pazirik. V c. B.C. About 5 x 4 in.

Fig. 63. Design on a sheath encasing a horse's tail in Mound 1, Pazirik. V c. B.C.

the creature, already discussed, on one of the Pazirik wall-hangings, for although anatomically it is more than half animal, spiritually it is altogether human. There is nothing bestial or primitive about it, and the impression it leaves is one of sophistication and elegance.

A hanging of a devotional character, likewise from Pazirik,

Fig. 61

provides a further example of the skill with which the nomads designed human representations. The textile measures some four yards by six, the design being repeated on it twice; it is carried out in coloured felts on an off-white felt ground.

Plate 30

The scene represents the Great Goddess seated on a throne of clearly local make since its turned legs closely resemble some found on furniture placed in the actual burials. However, the deity wears a robe more closely resembling a Chinese dress than an Altaian costume, nor do the rider's clothes or his features correspond to those of the nomads. The curious candelabra-like standard belonging to the goddess is, however, derived from an antler pattern, and the hanging is without doubt local both in manufacture and inspiration.

The profusion of decorated objects, whether of Scythian or Altaian origin, far surpasses, at any rate in quantity, anything produced by any ancient group of people of equivalent size. For this reason, quite apart from stylistic considerations and archæological evidence, it is evident that the work was carried out by the nomads themselves in the course of their daily life and not, as is sometimes suggested, by professional craftsmen working to their order in the more readily accessible urban centres. The Chinese writers noticed that among the Orkhan vassals of the Huns 'the women embroider in silk on leather and weave woollen stuffs; the men make bows and arrows, saddles and bridles, mould gold and iron for arms'. Much the same division of labour probably held good in Eurasia and the Pazirik finds show that almost every member of the tribe must have been skilled at some form of handiwork. Looking at their creations after a lapse of over two thousand years it seems difficult to deny them the title of artists. Yet critics such as David Sinor[31] consider their contribution to art 'very modest' when compared to 'the achievements of European, Chinese and Indian art'. This opinion is surely based on a false premise, since the Scythian and kindred tribes did not create a culture, but merely a style in art. It would be fairer to contrast their achievements with those of the Phœnicians, Etruscans or any other similar small and short-lived racial unit rather than to set them beside the great civilizations which were built up over centuries by a great body of people linked by national and religious ties.

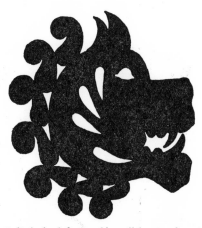

Fig. 64. A lion's head from a felt wall-hanging from Mound 1, Pazirik. V c. B.C. About 5 x 5 in.

The Scythian contribution to the world's store of master-pieces is far from negligible. Some of their metal-work is of perennial worth and certain of their single animal designs, such as the Kelermes leopard, the lion from a Pazirik wall-hanging or the lion from a Pazirik saddle-cloth can stand comparison with Picasso's illustrations to Buffon or with the animal draw-ings of any school of art. Though they did not enrich the world with any monumental works, the Scythians formed a bridge between the ancient world and Slavonic Russia, and they left behind them a style that influenced the development of several branches of European art. In addition, they succeeded in

Plate 9
Figs. 64, 65

creating a veritable people's art. This is a rare achievement.
Unlike a craft, which is in the main the product of skilled but
not especially vital professionals, and unlike a folk art, which is
maintained by able but unimaginative traditionalists, a people's
art is conceived and practised by an entire community. It has
been given to few groups of people to evolve an art of this type.
That the Scythian and kindred tribesmen succeeded in doing
so is shown by the objects which they took with them to their
graves.

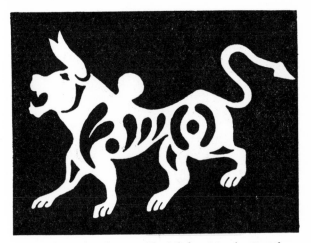

Fig. 65. A lion from a saddle-cloth from Mound 1, Pazirik.
V c B.C. Worked in felt and measuring about 9 x 6 in.

SOURCES

Numbers in parentheses refer to the Bibliography on p. 201.

1   Mongait (85), p. 98.

2   *Ibid.*, pp. 92–3. These excavations covered the years 1926–39.

3   Frankfort (11), p. 212.

4   Mongait (85), p. 117.

5 Pietrovsky (87), p. 8.

6 Frankfort (11), p. 115–16.

7 Vieyra (37), p. 11.

8 Piggott (21).

9 Mongait (85), pp. 116–20.

10 Ravdonikas (89), and Rudenko (91).

11 Zakharov (98), p. 227.

12 Turaev (72), p. 33.

13 Schefeld (50), p. 73, and Contenau (55).

14 Ghirshman (13), p. 106, fig. 48.

15 For illustration, see Minns (18), fig. 65.

16 Vieyra (37), Pl. 32.

17 Ghirshman (13), p. 108, fig. 48.

18 Frankfort (11), fig. 7e, p. 16.

19 Rostovtzeff (27), pp. 22–3.

20 Mongait (85), p. 98.

21 Zelenin (99), pp. 297–309.

22 For illustration, see Minns (18), fig. 146.

23 Marr and Smirnov (62).

24 Talbot Rice (23), Vol I.

25 Trever (35), pp. 33–4, Pl. 8–10.

26 Shilov, *Soobshcheniya Gosndarstvennovo Ermitaja IX,* Leningrad 1956, p. 41.

27 Salmony, *Antler and Tongue, an Essay on ancient Chinese symbolism and its implications.* Artibus Asiæ, Ascona, 1954. See fig. 23, p. 17.

28 Tarassuk (97) p. 25.

29 Salmony, *op. cit.,* p. 19. For illustration see fig. 9, p. 9.

30 Childe (7), fig. 26, No. 59.

31 Sinor (31), p. 90.

M

CHAPTER VI

The Scythian Legacy

THE SCYTHIANS VANISHED from the pages of history as abruptly as they had entered; it was as though they had fallen into a deep well, for though they themselves disappeared, very considerable ripples were left behind them. These spread over much of Europe, but it is scarcely surprising that the most profound of them formed over Russia, where their fluid out-lines were occasionally visible even in the present century. They survived most clearly in the peasant art, notably in embroideries, wood carvings, and in the pottery and toys which the peasants made for their own use on lines which often show little change from pagan times.

Far too scant attention has been paid to the history of the pagan Slavs who replaced the Scythians and Sarmatians in the European section of the Eurasian plain, and who succeeded in establishing there the foundations of the state which was eventually to play its part in history as the Russia of the Tsars. The centuries during which the country was gradually becoming unified and her culture was slowly evolving were hazardous and turbulent, for the inhabitants of southern Russia were in constant danger of attack from various nomadic tribes living to the east of them, who were gradually being forced westward from central or even from farther Asia.

After the Scythian collapse and the rise to power of the Sarmatians, life had marked time for a span; then, by about the second century A.D., trade within the country had revived. The impetus had come from the Sarmatians who, perhaps as a result of their eastern origin, shared the Siberian people's love of brilliant, scintillating colours and the Scythians' predilection for animal forms and precious materials, but who, at the same time, lacked the skill to satisfy these tastes. They were perforce obliged to turn to the Greek craftsmen of the northern Pontus for what they needed. In most cases, however, Hellenism reached them in a Scythian guise, that is to say, it implied for them rich-looking ornaments and luxurious jewels. Of a different temperament from the Scythians, with a less keen feeling for outline, and with their artistic judgment unformed by contacts with the Ancient Orient, the Sarmatians preferred a shimmering, opalescent surface to sinuous line, and an in-tricate polychrome effect to the light and play of rich metal and balanced design. Their taste bore the stamp of Minussinsk, the Altai and the Don, and they demanded from the Greek metal-workers objects in gold or bronze with brightly irides-cent surfaces and rich decoration.

The polychrome style was revived to satisfy these wishes. The Greek craftsmen set out to produce the desired effect by overlaying the metal ground of the ornament either with champlevé work, in accordance with which stones and enamel inlays were placed in prepared cavities, or with cloisonné, where tiny metal partitions separate the coloured paste or glass inlays; or again coloured stones and jewels were mounted in settings of metal wire. Many of the objects which were deco-rated in these ways retained the animal outlines which the Scythians had loved, but when the Goths invaded the land from the west, they brought new shapes with them, and these were soon added to the repertory. Thus new types of arms and jewellery were introduced into the area, and both the old and the new forms were decorated with polychrome work, regard-less of whether they were intended for use by the Sarmatians or the Goths. The latter were already fond of beast forms in art, and they were therefore attracted by the Scythian designs, but they had a particular liking for birds of prey. Under their in-fluence the stag began to lose its importance in the art of the area, its place being taken by the bird forms of Gothic art. But by that time the Pontic Greeks had themselves succumbed to the fascination of polychrome decoration, with the result that the style became as much the fashion with them as it was with the Sarmatians and the Goths. In each case, however, it continued to remain basically Scythian beneath the gay, super-imposed veneer.

During this period, the political situation in the south of Russia remained troubled and dangerous, and the Slav agri-culturists of the region continued to live in subservience, poverty and fear. They were primitive people and in constant want. Superstitions of every sort dominated their life. To ward off the ever impending evil they invented gods of every descrip-tion, erecting in their honour wooden idols and totem poles in the squares and market-places, propitiating the gods with offerings, and carving magical figures on the faces of rocks and the bark of trees. To safeguard themselves from the evil eye they hung tiny amulets of horses, birds and mugs on their chests. On their belts they wore a comb, as the Scythians had done before them, but they also generally carried an amulet of a bear, this animal having acquired considerable religious significance amongst them. Finally, there was added to this animal reper-tory sometime between the first and fifth centuries A.D. amulets such as crosses, triangles, rhomboids, circles and so on, all of which were in one way or another concerned with the solar cult that became extremely important after the fifth century. These symbols were placed on vessels and utensils, as much in order to serve as a protection as in an act of homage to the deity.

It was with inherent Russian ruthlessness that, by order of Vladimir, Grand Prince of Kiev, the pagan idols, totem poles and other articles of heathen worship were destroyed in the year 988, at the time of the country's conversion to Christianity. Nevertheless, the peasantry of the land continued to cling to their native traditions and beliefs with no less characteristic tenacity, and although all the tangible heathen monuments perished, far more of the discarded cult was preserved than is generally realized. Paganism itself continued to flourish unabated in much of the country till well into the twelfth century; it even survived into the nineteenth century here and there in the remoter regions of the land, and beside it many pre⁄Christian forms and symbols were preserved until the revolu⁄tion, in the shape of the toys the peasants made for their children. Most popular among these toys were wooden chariots and horses, which were in fact exact replicas, complete with solar symbols, of those which, in pagan times, had been thought to draw the sun daily across the firmament.

Among the various practices which the Slavs inherited from the Scythians, the most important consisted in the worship of their ancestors. In accordance with Scythian custom, they too buried their leaders in tombs equipped with all the essentials of life, and they also placed the dead man's wife, decked in her wedding dress, in his burial chamber, but they led her into it alive, there to meet her death. They raised mounds above these burials, offering sacrifices and holding tourneys and wakes on their summits. Each year, they foregathered again on the spot, to offer fresh sacrifices in memory of the dead. A Slav whose horse had been killed in battle outdid the Scythians in the honours which he paid to his dead mount, for he would have its body placed on a high platform, which was then covered by a mound as large as that built over a soldier's grave. It is like⁄wise probable that the Slav habit of placing a sword beside a newly⁄born boy and of seating the child on a horse on his third birthday also accorded with Scythian tradition.

It was during the fifth century A.D. that the people living in the south of Russia began to worship the sun. As a result the horse and cock, both of them solar symbols, became prominent in their art. The symbolic importance of the horse became even greater in the following century, when stables were built close to the solar temples to house the animals considered holy. Horses endowed with magical powers now found a place in the people's sagas, and were soon joined by the fire-bird and by cocks. The latter took the firmest hold on the people's imagina- tion, the form surviving longer in Slav art than any of the other ancient motifs, retaining its prominence throughout the Slav world right down to modern times, even if its meaning had been forgotten. The versions which appear in Russian and Balkan lace and embroideries trace their descent to the cocks of the Scythian Altai. Indeed the prototypes of all the later Slav renderings of this motif are to be found among the contents of Mounds 1 and 2 at Pazirik. The most interesting of the Pazirik

Fig. 25

versions are the two splendidly schematized silhouettes cut out of leather, which was then gilt, from Mound 1. In these a magnificently spirited and most sophisticated stylization is combined with an unexpected yet wholly harmonious natural- ism. The effect is achieved by the inclusion of the untidy little feathers which grow on the back of a cock's legs. The blend of abstraction and veracity is also characteristic of Russian decora- tive art, and designs which come very close to the Altaian examples were produced early in the present century, long before the discovery of Pazirik, by the distinguished 'World of Art' artist, Goncharova, working in a traditional 'Russian' style.[1] The antler-like element in the Pazirik cock's combs likewise survive in Slav art, and the kinship remains clearly marked in other respects.

The Russian Slavs gradually combined the solar cult with that of the Great Goddess, adding solar symbols to those which had long been hers. They venerated her with no less devotion than the Scythians. The creed took especially deep root in the heavily wooded regions of Russia, where the peasants paid homage to the Great Goddess in sacred groves and at spring heads. The practice actually persisted in some out-of-the-way places until the outbreak of the last war. Those participating in the rite liked to find a birch tree standing alone in a clearing; they would choose it to personify the goddess, decking it in a woman's dress and hanging on one of its branches the canonical towel, embroidered in red with the figure of the goddess, her attendants and attributes. When no such tree could be found, a young girl with branches of birch twined in her hair was placed in the centre of the clearing and the towel was hung on a convenient bough. The people then formed a ring round the goddess's representative, dancing in a circle and stamping to simulate the sound of running horses.

The ceremonial towel ranked as a family heirloom. It had been worked by an ancestress and, together with the family's icons, it was numbered among the household's most treasured

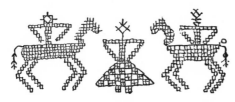

Fig. 66. A XIXth-c. Lithuanian peasant towel embroidered with the figures of the Great Goddess flanked by mounted chieftains. Musée de l'Homme, Paris.

possessions. The towel's designs closely followed early proto-types, with the goddess invariably forming its main motif. She often appears in the same pose as that in which she is shown on Scythian metal-work, being generally flanked either by two princely horsemen, who sometimes have birch twigs twined in their hair and hold offerings, or by mounted priests, the reins of whose horses are firmly grasped by the all-controlling deity. The background is filled in with various solar symbols such as cocks, horses, ducks, hares and fire-birds.

Fig. 66

On becoming engaged, a Slav girl was expected to work a ceremonial towel of this sort as a gift to her groom. She also had to make her wedding dress, embroidering it with designs which conformed to tradition. In Yugoslavia in particular, many of the costumes still being worn today retain details which can be traced back to Scythian dress, even though the majority have lost their original shapes. In some cases the patterns have become distorted simply as a result of the passage of time, representational forms having been transformed into geometric ones; in other instances change seems to have been intentional, ideograms having been substituted for pagan symbolism at a time when the latter was being fiercely eradicated by the Christian clergy. In Russia, however, some of the patterns have retained their original names, and these give a clue to their meaning by disclosing that certain designs, which are now abstract, are known as the goat, the cock, the calf-eye, and more significant still, the antler pattern.

Scythian influence can also be detected in the sculptured decorations which appear on Russian churches of late medieval date. They are to be most clearly observed in the series that adorns the façades of the twelfth- and thirteenth-century churches of the Vladimir-Suzdal district, notably the Church of the Intercession of the Holy Virgin at Nerl and the Cathedral of St. George at Uriev Polsky.[2] On both of these buildings curious and enchanting beasts of a rather heraldic type stand amidst a profusion of Christian and other symbols. These delightful creatures have long puzzled art historians. Some have ascribed them to the influence of Christian Georgia and Armenia, whilst others have traced them to the Roman-esque art of western Europe. The manner of their disposition on the walls is western rather than eastern in conception, but the Christian elements and the general style are derived either direct from Byzantium or from Armenia and Georgia. The animals themselves, however, bear a very close connection with many of the creatures evolved by Scythian designers. They represent indeed a revival of local forms which were reanimated and transformed into something temperamentally wholly new by the Christian artists of the region.

Until the westernizing reforms of Peter the Great altered the course of the country's development, Russian decorative art retained a great many Scythian mannerisms. Although zoomorphic junctures and stag forms were abandoned, many bird patterns persisted, appearing as decorations on various examples of metal-work, ceramics, needlework and firearms. Some domestic utensils, and more particularly spoons and wine-tasters, retained Scythian shapes and continued to display the stud and arrow-head motifs which are so characteristic of Scythian ornamentation.

During the Sarmatian and the pagan Slav period of Russian history commercial relations were established between the people of the Black Sea area and those living in the Baltic lands. Goods were transported from the one region to the other along the great rivers which intersect Russia. This trade gradually came to be controlled by the Germanic peoples who had followed the Goths in their advance into the Bosphoran zone. Many of these hangers-on settled on the banks of the Dniestr and in the northern Pontus, but they kept in regular touch with their homelands. Artistic trends, objects and coins now travelled up the great rivers together with bales and sacks of goods, and it was in this way that designs which were still basically Scythian, though transformed by the Pontic artists to conform to Sarmato-Gothic taste, filtered into Scandinavia and northern Germany.

The influence is reflected in Scandinavian art from a very early date. It can be discerned in the late-Celtic period of its history, in objects dating from about the first to the second centuries A.D. It appears for example in an imported vessel, the magnificently ornamented great silver cauldron from Gundestrup[3] in Jutland, measuring twenty-eight inches across. Some of the animal motifs which decorate it are very close to Scythian work, and the inclusion of imaginary beasts and elephants points unquestionably to definite eastern connections.

Scythian again is the disposition of the scenes. In one register a row of mounted soldiers is shown advancing towards the right, in a lower one they march towards the left. As has been noted, this was a favourite Scythian arrangement and it must surely have reached Scandinavia from the south of Russia, even though Shetelig favours the alternative suggestion that the cauldron may have been carried northward by Celts living on the Danube.

The commerce between Scandinavia and south Russia was interrupted in the fourth century when the Huns advanced towards the Black Sea from the east, evicting the Goths and isolating the area. Nevertheless, the Scytho-Sarmatian style probably continued to influence the decorations produced in Scandinavia between about A.D. 450 and 600, even though Shetelig[4] argues against this view, firstly because the gap between the heyday of Scythia's art and the dawn of the migration style in Scandinavia was considerable, and secondly because of the absence of stags in Germanic animal art, which was the main source of the Scandinavian style. He omits, however, to take into account the art of the Sarmatians or to consider the persistence of many Scytho-Sarmatian elements in the art of the early Slavs of Russia. It is impossible to disregard the effect this must have had on the northern artists. Shetelig ascribes much in Scandinavia to the influence of Roman industrial art, and to a lesser extent, to Germanic animal art. The latter had itself received valuable contributions from the Scytho-Sarmatian school,[5] the Hallstatt and La Tène Celts having served as intermediaries between the two, a fact which must have attuned the Scandinavians to respond sympathetically to similar trends coming to them direct from southern Russia. A very individual style resulted in Scandinavia from the blend of these various elements. It served as a basis for the somewhat later Viking art of the region, and this in turn was eventually carried to Britain, where it expressed itself with the utmost felicity in Celtic and Saxon carving and jewellery.

The Scytho-Sarmatian elements which survived in the art of the Slavs once again regained their hold on Scandinavian artists when contacts with the south of Russia were intensified by the Vikings, who established themselves there in the ninth century. They even settled in the region of the Volga and the Caspian, where Scythian art forms continued to flourish in an even purer form. Small-scale objects, such as the bronze plaques from Borre in Norway, show this very clearly both as regards the repertory of the animals that appear upon them—

Plate 42

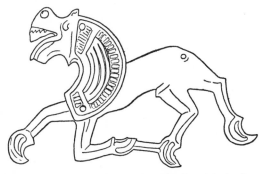

Fig. 67. Silver plaque of Slav workmanship from Martinovka, near Kiev. VI c. A.D.

stags, griffins and imaginary creatures—and in the style. Even the muscle markings which are included are clearly derived from the Scythian dot and comma convention. The same influence is also evident in large-scale work, notably the animal figureheads on the Viking ships, such as those from Oseberg and Gökstadt, placed there to ward off the evil eye. The Gökstadt horse fits into the Scythian frame particularly well. It is in the same style as the Borre plaques, thus differing slightly from the more ornate and florid Oseberg manner. Its ancestry can be traced back to a bronze horse from Kerch of mid-Scythian date. The influence might have come direct from southern Russia, being tempered on the way by the Slavs who

Plate 43

Plate 44

Fig. 67

Plate 45

Fig. 68

created works similar to those found in a hoard of the sixth century A.D. from Martinovka, near Kiev,[6] or it may have followed a more devious course, travelling by way of Hallstatt. It can be seen there in a flagon dating from the fourth or third century B.C., found at Basse-Yutz in Lorraine. Though of Persian shape, the bronze handle in the form of a wolf is essentially Scythian in character. By the migration period this style had in its turn changed to the heavier and more ornate form which is admirably expressed in a bronze ornament of the sixth century A.D. from Hungary.

Somewhat similar Scytho-Sarmatian trends even penetrated as far as Britain. The style was on the one hand carried to her shores by the Vikings and came on the other by the more circuitous route across Germany. Once again southern Russia served as the starting point, for when the Goths fled from the Pontus to attack and overrun much of south-western Europe, they carried with them their polychrome jewellery and metal-work, disseminating it, together with the Scytho-Sarmatian elements on which it was based, throughout many outlying regions. In this way the animal style was revived first in Romania, then in Austria, then in the Rhineland, whence it travelled, along with other elements, to England.

The Scytho-Sarmatian influence was particularly marked in central Europe. This was perhaps due to the infiltration of Eurasian elements into the area at the time of the late Hallstatt and early La Tène periods, that is to say from about 500 B.C. onwards. The Hallstatt Celts lived the same sort of life as did the Eurasian nomads, and a Hallstatt sword in the Natur-historisches Museum in Vienna[7] shows that their profusely trimmed trousers were very like those worn by the Scyths on the Chertomlyk vessel, whilst their tail-coats seem to have resembled those that Radlov found at Katanda. Jacobstahl regards the area and the people as 'the westernmost outpost of the vast Eurasian belt',[8] and indeed Eurasian elements are constantly cropping up in their objects. Rows of beasts walk in single file, though in only one direction, along the rims of countless of their bronze vessels, beading and hatching are regular decorative motifs, pyramids, circles and other Scythian patterns often recur, and the Great Goddess flanked by two beasts is a familiar figure. Even a migration period variant from as far west as Amiens, where it figures characteristically on a horse-trapping, keeps very close to Eurasian versions.

Plate 41

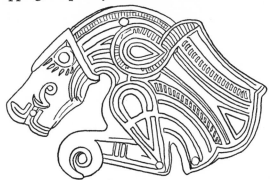

Fig. 68. Bronze horse of the VI c. A.D. from Hungary. Budapest National Museum.

Scythian influence first made its mark in Hungary round about the year 500 B.C., when the foremost wave of Scythians penetrated to the area. Its reflection is mirrored in a number of late Hallstatt works. The connection is not only to be noted in stylistic affinities, however; it is confirmed by archæological evidence collected during the last forty years or so. This shows that the western Scyths and eastern Celts were in some sort of touch with one another. Thus, in 1910, Spitzin[9] discovered at Nemirovo in Podolia in western Russia Scythian objects lying with fragments of typical Hallstatt pottery; Danilevski found the same when excavating various sites in the district of Kiev and along the Dniepr, and Bobrinsky unearthed La Tène as well as Hallstatt ware during several excavations conducted within the limits of the Dniepr. Conversely, Párducz, excavating at Szentes-Vekerzug in Hungary as recently as 1952[10], encountered a most complex state of affairs. The Vekerzug burials cover a large area and are of a mixed character. Many contained horse burials which include horse-trappings; in some there also lay mirrors, trefoil arrow-heads and other Scythian objects, whilst in others nothing Scythian was found. The same situation existed at a number of allied sites such as Egreskáta, Mátraszele and Chotin. At all of these the Scythians and Celts appear to have intermixed, and the same seems to have happened in certain regions of Transylvania. It is still impossible to draw a clear distinction in these mixed burial grounds between the tombs of each group, but Párducz feels convinced that the burials show 'quite definite signs of Scythian customs'. Matsulevich[11] likewise, when describing a grave of a 'barbarian king' found in eastern Europe, draws attention to some harness ornaments belonging to it. The most interesting were snake-shaped but had the heads of fish-birds. They resembled on the one hand some Scythian examples from Kerch and on the other some fibulæ of the fifth century A.D. found on the Oise in France. The Balkan burials thus provide a link between Scythian Kerch and Merovingian France.

In the various areas within the sphere of the Hallstatt and La Tène cultures the art of the migration period is strongly linked. Although it developed in each region along independent lines, it yet converged at times to borrow some motif or detail from the main stream. Such features were often retained virtually unaltered for centuries, and at times passed to a neighbour, in whose hands the patterns frequently survived unchanged. Sometimes, however, they developed into independent, thoroughly alien variants. Nowhere can the interrelationship which binds them be more clearly perceived than in the recurrence throughout the entire area of the large beaked bird motif. Even a cursory glance at its distribution reveals its astonishing persistence and penetration. There is thus a startling connection, to which Rostovtzeff has drawn attention,[12] between a magnificent gold and polychrome bird of Siberian origin and the birds forming part of the fifth-century A.D. Petroasa horde. The former shows an eagle or other large beaked bird devouring a stag; the latter, and especially the large bird in gold and polychrome work, is closely similar to it. The Goths' fondness for birds of prey played its part in preserving this large beaked, round-eyed Scythian bird motif, the creature remaining popular throughout much of western Europe for many centuries. Thus a very early Scythian version in bone from Kelermes reappears in the Frankish world many years later almost unaltered, whether produced in heavy bronze or in delicate enamel.

Plate 46

Plate 47

Plates 48–50

One of the latest, and possibly most exquisite large beaked birds comes from far-distant England, on the purse lid from the treasure of Sutton Hoo in Suffolk. The treasure is dated to A.D. 655–656, and the bird, which is about to pounce on a duck, already shows slight touches of the elongation which was later to become characteristic of English painting and sculpture. Yet it adheres remarkably closely to the Frankish versions, and through them to the Scythian originals. The Norse character is perhaps rather more to the fore in some of the other enamel ornaments attached to the purse, but the Celto-Scythian element is indisputably the most important in the bird. The disk affixed to the boss of the Sutton Hoo shield represents a two-headed creature which has much in sympathy with works of the mid-Scythian period and the Basse-Yutz jug handle. One of its extremities is a forcefully stylized version of the large beaked bird, but by means of a somewhat clumsy and simplified zoomorphic juncture, its back turns into a dragon's head, which can to some extent be paralleled by a carving from Mound 2 at Pazirik.[13] The general treatment of the ornament also bears certain similarities to the Hungarian horse of the migration period.

Plate 52

Plate 51

Plate 45

Fig. 68

A resemblance to Scythian art can often be recognized in the sculptures and illuminations of the Celtic school in Britain. The Cross at Papil on the Isle of Burra in the Shetlands,[14] now dated to the eighth century or before, includes a lion characterized by the alert bearing, rounded eye and muscle markings of a Scythian beast; the calf of St. Luke from the Durrow Gospels[15] shows the same markings, for even though they are transformed into decorative features the dot and comma origin of the pattern is still recognizable. The marking may have been transmitted to England from a Hallstatt base, since it frequently figures in the pottery of the later phase of that culture, as, for example, on the Scythian-looking beasts decorating the clay flask found at Matzhausen, now in Berlin.[16]

Fig. 69

The cross of Abbotsford, in the Museum of Antiquities in Edinburgh, shows an animal again marked by a number of Scythian features. Thus the creature's tail terminates, by means of a zoomorphic juncture, in a snake's head; its pointed feet trace

Plates 24, 28
Fig. 67

their descent back to the Kul Oba and Zoldhalompuszta stags, by way of the Slav plaques from Martinovka; furthermore the ridge along its back indicating three-dimensional relief, the comma-like lines outlining the face, the oval eye and pointed ear can all be paralleled in Eurasia.

These resemblances could be multiplied time and again, but the likeness appears at its most striking in a group of eleventh-century Saxon stone slabs. One of these, originally in St. Paul's churchyard and now in the Guildhall Museum,

Plate 54

London,[17] shows a stag of wholly Scythian character. Its pose had not greatly altered in the fifteen hundred years which had elapsed since the Scythians first made the motif their own. Its muscle markings, which date back to Alaça Hüyük, two thousand five hundred years earlier, are still in place though somewhat altered in shape, but even more important is the similarity in feeling. The man who carved this stone must have felt the wind blowing westward from southern Russia across

Scandinavia, wafting a last flicker of inspiration from a long-dead Scythian source.

The western animal style which the Scythians helped to form served in its turn as a spring-board for Romanesque sculptors and early medieval illuminators, but their art, though having its roots set so far back in antiquity, expressed the ancient formulas in an entirely novel way. The new style discarded all trace of the Scythian, yet it is highly probable that animals

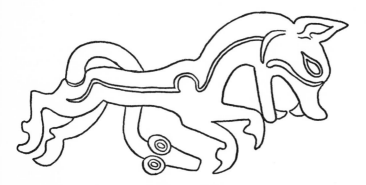

Fig. 69. An animal from the Abbotsford cross, formerly at Woodwray, Forfarshire.

would not have played so large a part in the art of early Europe had not the Scythians lived first, to evolve an animal art and to develop an interest in and an understanding of animal forms in so many regions of the western world.

In the fifth and fourth centuries B.C. west and east converged at Pazirik, at any rate in so far as imported articles were concerned, for it was from this area that both western and Scythian trends percolated to China. Contacts between China and the eastern nomads had indeed been established at an early date, and were maintained by trade and exchanges of gifts, the Chinese presenting fine lacquer and exquisite silks to the nomadic

N

chieftains whom they wished to propitiate. The Scythian objects which have been found in the Ordos and as far within China's borders as Uliafu in the province of Chensu may have been gifts offered in return by the Scyths, though it is also possible, indeed on the whole more likely, that they were acquired by individual Chinese.[18] Yet the two peoples do not seem to have had many common interests or tastes, for although they occasionally borrowed a motif or a detail from each other's repertory, the influence which they exercised over one another was largely superficial. Thus the stamped copper plaque from Mound 2 at Pazirik bearing confronted animals is but a rare instance of the Chinese element in Altaian art, and there is singularly little trace of this element in Scythia. Objects such as the pre-Han mirror discovered in Mound 6 at Pazirik should be clearly distinguished as imports.

Fig. 70

If the nomads did not often see through Chinese eyes, they nevertheless succeeded in leaving their mark on the art of the Ordos and the Hunan. There, from as early as the fourth till as late, at any rate, as the first century B.C., bronze and silver plaques occur, bearing stags, mules, horses, leopards or tigers, either galloping or in a recumbent position with movement arrested. They frequently show very close affinities with the somewhat earlier Scythian works and there is every reason to believe that these should be regarded as their prototypes. Other objects reflect the style of Pazirik and Siberia, whilst a bronze plaque in the British Museum displays a tiger which is clearly related to those which adorn the face of the Basadar coffin. This Chinese beast of prey carries a ram, which is in turn closely allied to the bone and wood carvings of Kelermes and Pazirik. Many plaques were decorated with animal forms which assume the familiar shape of a horizontal B. These too serve to show that throughout the latter half of the first millennium B.C. the nomads of Siberia must have been in regular touch with the people living on the fringes of China.

Plates 61–2

Plate 56

Plates 36–7

Plates 53, 56

Yet the Eurasian influence was not confined solely to the outlying districts of that great empire—it made itself felt in China proper, even though its role at first proved mainly in, direct, and consisted primarily in transmitting to the Orient certain of the animal forms which had been evolved in the

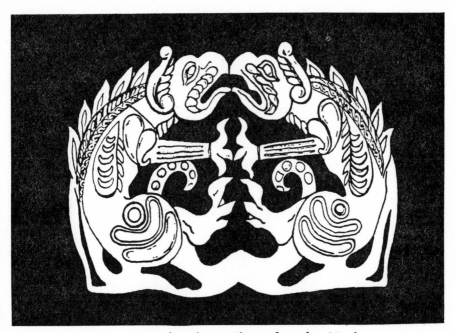

Fig. 70. Copper plaque showing Chinese influence from Mound 2, Pazirik. V c. B.C. About 4½ x 3½ in.

west. Its effect is especially marked in the Hunan where the art of the Chu age, which largely contained animal motifs, came to include many western beasts, such as stylized tigers, horned lions and eagle-headed griffins, that can have reached China only from the Middle East, where they are to be found regularly in Assyrian and Sumerian art of an earlier date. Even the Han dragon, though regarded to-day as a specifically

Chinese creature, was probably evolved from blending the tiger and the phœnix, a process for which the Persian Simurg may have been responsible. The square or round patterns with which the Chinese covered the bodies of their bronze animals were similarily almost certainly derived from the dot, comma and half-moon markings which the Eurasian nomads used with such astonishing frequency, and which reappeared much later as a favourite motif on Turkish textiles.

Under the Hans, the influence of Siberian art of the Scythian type became for a time so forceful that some of the oriental bronze plaques scarcely differed in arrangement and form from the nomadic works,[19] whilst the Chinese dragon became twisted into an altogether Scythian posture, its head being turned in one direction and its body in another.[20] At much the same time oriental metal-workers began to stylize the tails and extremities of many of their beasts in accordance with the convention characteristic of Altaian and Scythian art, and the pole and furniture finials which had flourished in Egypt, the ancient Orient, Siberia and Scythia since early prehistoric times appeared in China. It was thus that the style which crystallized in Eurasia penetrated at one time or another both to the east and to the west, where it came to serve as the starting point for more than one new fashion in the decorative arts of many widely separated lands.

Plates 57–60

SOURCES

Numbers in parentheses refer to the Bibliography on p. 201.

1 Notably in the setting of Act III for Diaghilev's ballet, *Coq d'Or*.

2 For illustrations, see Buxton (5), Pl. 8–15.

3 Falk and Shetelig (10), P. 31, p. 189.

4 *Ibid.*, p. 294.

5 Picton (20), Ch. I.

6 Grabar (79), p. 53.

7 Jacobstahl (16), Pl. 60, No. 96.

8 *Ibid.*, p. 162.

9 Makarenko (61), pp. 22–3.

10 Párducz (65), pp. 25–89.

11 Matsulevich (63).

12 Rostovtzeff (27), p. 186.

13 Rudenko (49), Pl. XXVIII.

14 Romilly, Allen (1), fig. 130, p. 359.

15 *Ibid.*, fig. 129, p. 358.

16 Jacobstahl (16), fig. 402.

17 Talbot Rice (24), p. 44.

18 Tolmacheff (71), p. 250–8.

19 Tibor Horvath (34). Plate 4 shows a tiger attacking an argall, of Siberian workmanship of the third to second century B.C.; Plate 5, a Sin-yuan Ordos bronze and silver plaque of the second to first century B.C., shows a tiger attacking a deer. These two bear a striking resemblance to each other.

20 Rostovtzeff (28), fig. 34.

Major Burials of the Scythians and Kindred Nomads

KUBAN GROUP

Elizavetovskaya Stanitza (V–IVc. B.C.).
Karagodenashkh (first half of IIIc. B.C.).
Kelermes (VII–VIc. B.C.).
Kostromskaya Stanitza (VII–VIc. B.C.).
Kurdzhips Barrows (IV–IIIc. B.C.).

Marjevskaya Stanitza (IVc. B.C.).
Seven Brothers Barrows (very early Vc. B.C.).
Ulski Barrows (VIc. B.C.).
Urupskaya Stanitza (IVc. B.C.).

TAMAN GROUP

Bolshaya Blisnitza (Great Twin) Barrows (IVc. B.C.).
Lake Zukur Barrows (Vc. B.C.).

Phanagoria Barrows (late IVc. B.C.).
Taman Barrows (last quarter of IVc. B.C.).
Vasjurin Barrows (early IIIc. B.C.).

CRIMEAN GROUP

Ak Metchet (VI–Vc. B.C.).
Altin Oba (early V—late IV c. B.C.).
Dört Oba (III c. B.C.).
El Tegen (Nymphæum) Second half IV c. B.C.).
Kara Kiat (Simferopol) (IIIc. B.C.).

Krim Estate (V–IV c. B.C.).
Kul Oba (early V—late IV c. B.C.).
Patiniotti (end of IV c. B.C.).
Temir Gora, near Kerch (VIIc. B.C.).
Tsarsky Kurgan (early V–late IV c. B.C.).
Salgir (III c. B.C.).

DNIEPR GROUP (mainly north of Perekop and along the river's left bank)

Alanovskaya Blisnitza (mid IVc. B.C.).
Alexandropol (mid IVc. B.C.).
Baby Kurgan (IV–IIIc. B.C.).
Bashmatski Kurgan (IIIc. B.C.).
Chertomlyk (IVc. B.C.).
Chmyrev Kurgan (V–IVc. B.C.).
Deev Kurgan (IVc. B.C.).
Dergaws (mid IVc. B.C.).

Kamennaya Mogila (IIIc. B.C.).
Lemeshovsky Kurgan (mid IVc. B.C.).
Malaya Lepaticha (mid IVc. B.C.).
Melgunov Barrows (VII—VIc. B.C.).
Mordvinov Barrows (mid IVc. B.C.).
Nicopol Barrows (mid IVc. B.C.).
Ogüz Barrows (latter half IIc. B.C.).
Ostraya Mogila (VI–Vc. B.C.).

DNIEPR GROUP—*cont.*

Raskopana Barrows (IV–IIIc. B.C.).
Rhyzhanovka (IVc. B.C.).
Seregozy Barrows (V–IVc. B.C.).
Shulgovka, near Melitopol (mid IVc. B.C.).
Solokha (not prior to mid IVc. B.C.).

Tolstiya Mogily (mid IVc. B.C.).
Tsymbalka (IVc. B.C.).
Verchni Rogastchik (mid IVc. B.C.).
Znamenka (IVc. B.C.).

DON GROUP

Elizavetovskaya Stanitza (V–IIIc. B.C.).
Five Brothers.

Novocherkask Treasure (Ic. B.C.–Ic. A.D.).
Voronezh Barrows (late IVc.–IIIc. B.C.).

KIEV GROUP

Berestniaga (late IVc. B.C.).
Bobritza (late IVc. B.C.).
Cherkask group (VI–Vc. B.C.).
Cholodny Yar (VIc. B.C.).
Galushchino (Vc. B.C.).
Iljinets (IVc. B.C.).
Litoi Kurgan (VIc. B.C.).
Martonosha (first half of VIc. B.C.).
Novossel (IVc. B.C.).
Ostraya Mogila and Kanevich group (VI–Vc. B.C.).

Perepiatchina (Vc. B.C.).
Raigorod (III–IIc. B.C.).
Sachnovka (IVc. B.C.).
Shkvola group in the Zvenigorod district (VIc. B.C.).
Smela district (VI–IIIc. B.C.).
Snosk Borovski (late IVc. B.C.).
Turji (Vc. B.C.).
Zabotin group (VIc. B.C.).
Zurovka and Kapitonovka (VIc. B.C.).

POLTAVA GROUP (*closely akin to* KIEV GROUP)

Akjutinsk burials (IVc. B.C.–Ic. A.D.).

Volkovsk group (III–Ic. B.C.).

VOLGA GROUP

Astrakhan group (V–IIc. B.C.).

Samara group (V–IIc. B.C.).

URAL GROUP

Bish Oba.

Orenburg.

The Scythians

ALTAI GROUP

Başadar (Frozen burials) (VI–III c. B.C.).
Katanda (Frozen burials) (V–IVc. B.C.).
Kurai.

Pazirik (Frozen burials) (V–IVc. B.C.).
Shibe (IV–IIIc. B.C.).
Tuekt (Mid VI c. B.C.).

NORTHERN MONGOLIA

Noin Ula (Ic. A.D.).

GERMANY

Plohmühlen (V–IVc. B.C.).

Vettersfeld (early Vc. B.C.).

HUNGARY

Tapioszentmarton (Vc. B.C.).

Zoldhalompuszta (Vc. B.C.).

ROMANIA

Boureni (late IV–IIIc. B.C.)
Cuciurul Mare (late IV–IIIc. B.C.).

Satu Mare (late IV–IIIc. B.C.).

Bibliography

THE LITERATURE ON SCYTHIA and the Scythians is far richer than is generally supposed. The essential reference works in the English language are: M. Rostovtzeff, *Iranians and Greeks in south Russia*, Oxford, 1922; and E. H. Minns, *Scythians and Greeks*, Cambridge, 1913, both of which contain well-nigh comprehensive bibliographies. S. I. Rudenko's, *Kulturnoe naselenie gornovo Altaya v Skifskoe vremia*, USSR Academy of Science, Moscow, 1953, is scarcely less indispensable. All the Pazirik line illustrations are drawn from this book. It also contains an extensive bibliography, though one which is mainly concerned with the Siberian region rather than with Scythia proper. The writer is greatly indebted to these scholars, for this book could hardly have been written without frequent reference to their works.

A great many articles dealing both with the Scythian and the kindred tribes have appeared since the revolution in numerous Soviet publications, but it has not proved possible to establish a comprehensive list of them. It is hoped, however, that the following bibliography, though far from complete will, if used in conjunction with those compiled by Rostovtzeff, Minns and Rudenko, provide a helpful basis for readers wishing to pursue the subject further than has proved possible in this small volume.

Abbreviations

SA	Sovetskaya Archeologia
TR AS	Trudi Arkheologicheskovo Siezda
IAK	Izvestia Arkheologicheskoi Komisii
IGAIMK or GAIMK	(Izvestia) Gosudarstvennoi Akademii Materialnoi Kulturi
AN	Akademia Nauk
KSIIMK	Kratkie Soobshchenia o dokladach polevich issle-dovani Instituta Istorii Materialnoi Kulturi
MIA	Materiali i issledovaniya po arkheologii SSSR
RANION	Rosiiskaya Assotsiatsia Nauchno-Issledovatelskich Institutov Obshestvennich Nauk
M	Moscow
L	Leningrad
ML	Moscow-Leningrad
ESA	Eurasia Septentrionalis Antiqua.

English

1   ALLEN, ROMILLY J., *Early Christian Symbolism*, London, 1887.

2   ARNE, T. T., 'Luristan and the West', ESA, No. IX.

3   ATKINSON, R. J. & S. Piggott, 'The Torrs Chamfrein', *Archaeologia* London, 1955.

4   BOROVKA, G., *Scythian Art*, London, 1928.

5   BUXTON, J. R., *Russian Mediaeval Architecture*, London, 1937.

6   CHILDE, GORDON V., 'The socketed celt in Upper Eurasia', *Report of the Institute of Archaeology*, X, 1954.

7   *New light on the most ancient East*, London, 1952.

8   DALTON, O. M., *The Treasure of the Oxus*, British Museum, 1926.

9   ELLSWORTH HUNTINGDON, *The Pulse of Asia*, Boston, 1919.

10   FALK and SHETELIG, *Scandinavian Archaeology*, Cambridge, 1931.

11   FRANKFORT, H., *The Art and Architecture of the Ancient Orient,* Pelican Art History, London, 1954.

12   FRAZER, J. G., *The Golden Bough,* abridged edition, London, 1952.

13   GHIRSHMAN, R., *Iran*, Pelican book.

14   GOLOMSTOK, E. A., 'The Pazirik burials of the Altai', *American Journal of Archaeology*, 1933, Vol. 37, No. I.

15   *Herodotus*, Rawlinson's translation.

16   JACOBSTAHL, P., *Early Celtic Art*, Oxford, 1944.

17   KENDRICK, T., *History of the Vikings.*

18   MINNS, E. H., *Scythians and Greeks*, Cambridge, 1913.
19   *The Art of the Northern Nomads*, 1942.

20   PICTON, H., *Early German Art and its Origins*, Batsford, 1939.

21   PIGGOTT, S., Article in *The Listener*, 10 November 1955.

22   POPE, A. U., *A Survey of Persian Art,* Oxford, 1932, Vol. I.

23   RICE, D. TALBOT, 'Achæmenid Jewelry', *Survey of Persian Art,* Oxford, 1932, Vol. I.
24   *English Art 871–1100,* Oxford, 1952.

25   RIPLEY, W. Z., *Races of Europe*, London.

26   ROSS, D., AND SKRINE, E. H., *The Heart of Asia.*

27   ROSTOVTZEFF, M., *Iranians and Greeks in south Russia*, Oxford, 1922.
28   *Central Asia, Russia and the animal style*, Skythica I, Prague, 1923.

29   SALMONY, A., 'An unknown Scythian find in Novocherkask', *ESA,* No. X.

30 SHETELIG, H. S., 'Norse style of ornamentation in the Viking settlements', *Acta Arch.,* Stockholm, Vol. XIX, 1948.

31 SINOR, D., *Orientalism and History,* Cambridge, 1954.

32 *Sutton Hoo ship burial,* The British Museum, 1951.

33 TALLGREN, 'Caucasian Monuments', ESA, No. V. 1930.

34 TIBOR HÓRVATH, *The Art of Asia,* Budapest.

35 TREVER, C., *Excavations in Mongolia,* Leningrad, 1932.

36 VAN LE COQ, A., *Buried Treasures of Chinese Turkestan,* London, 1928.

37 VIEYRA, M., *Hittite Art,* London, 1955.

38 XENOPHON, *Cyropaedia.*

39 YETTS, P., 'The horse as a factor in early Chinese history', ESA, No. XX, and LLEWELLYN, B., *China's Court and Concubines,* London, 1956.

40 'Discoveries of the Kozlov expedition', *Burlington Magazine,* April 1926.

German

41 FETTICH, N., 'Zum Problem des Ungarländischen Stils', ESA, No. IX.
42 *Bronzeguss und Nomaden Kunst,* Prague, 1929.

43 GRIESSMAIER, V., *Sammlung Baron Eduard von der Heyat,* Vienna, 1936.

44 JETTMAR, K., 'Blonde und Blauäugige in Zentralasien', *Umschau,* No. 17, 1951.

45 MANĆAR, F., 'Caucasus-Luristan', ESA, No. IX, 1934.

46 MARTIN, J., 'Die Skythen in Schlesien', *Schlesiens Vorzeit in Bild und Schrift,* 1928.

47 RADLOV, W., *Aus Sibirien,* Leipzig, 1884.

48 RAVDONIKAS, W., *Die Normanen des Wiking Zeit und das Ladogagebiet,* Stockholm, 1930.

49 RUDENKO, S. I., *Der zweite Kurgan von Pazyryk,* Berlin, 1952.

50 SCHEFELD, K., 'Der Skythische Tierstil in süd Russland', ESA, No. XII, 1938.

51 VASMER, M., *Untersuchungen über die ältesten Wohnsitze des Slaven. Die Iranien in süd Russland,* Leipzig, 1923.

French

52 ARENDT, W. W., 'Sur l'apparition de l'étrier chez les Scythes', ESA, No. IX.

53 BASHMAKOFF, A. A., *Cinquante siècles d'évolution éthnique autour de la mer Noire,* Paris, 1937.

54 BÖKÖNII, S., Les chevaux Scythiques de Szentes-Vekerzug 2. Les fouilles de 1952–53, *Arch. Hung.* IV, 1954.

55 CONTENAU, G., *Manuel d'archéologie orientale,* 1937.

56 FETTICH, N., *Le trouvail Scythe de Zöldhalompuszta,* Budapest, 1928.

57 GRIASNOV, M., *Le kourgane de Pasyryk,* ML, 1931.

58 GROUSSET, R., *L'Empire des steppes,* Paris, 1939.

59 HEINKEL, A., *Antiquités de la Sibèrie Occidentale,* Helsingfors, 1894.

60 Hermitage Museum publication: *La réconstitution des couleurs primitives d'un tapis de Noïn Ula,* L. 1937.

61 MAKARENKO, N., 'La civilisation des Scythes de Hallstatt', ESA, No. V.

62 MARR, H., AND SMIRNOV, J., *Les Vichaps,* Leningrad, 1931.

63 MATSULEVICH, L. A., *Une sépulture d'un roi Barbare en Europe orientale*, Leningrad, 1934.

64 MORGAN, J. DE, *Préhistoire orientale*, Vol. III, 1927.

65 PÁRDUCZ, M., Le cimetière Hallstattien de Szentes-Vekerzug 2. Les fouilles de 1952–53, *Acta. Arch. Hung.*, 1954.

66 PELLIOT, P., *Quelques reflexions sur l'art sibérien et l'art chinois à propos de bronze de la collection David-Weill*, Paris, 1929.

67 PIETROWSKY, B. B., SCHULTZE, P. N., AND GOLOVKINA, V. A., TOLSTOY, S. P., *Ourartou, Néapolis des Scythes, Kharezm*, L'Orient ancient illustré, No. 8, Paris.

68 REINACH, S., KONDAKOV AND TOLSTOY, *Antiquités de la Russie méri-dionale*, Paris, 1892.

69 ROSTOVTZEFF, M., *L'art gréco-sarmate et l'art chinois à l'époque des Hans*, Paris.

70 'Le culte de la Grande Déesse dans la Russie méridionale', *Revue des études Grecques*, Vol. 32.

71 TOLMACHEV, V., 'Les antiquités des Scythes en Chine', ESA, No. IX.

72 TURAEV, B., 'Objets egyptiens et égyptisants trouvés en Russie méri-nionale', *Russkaya Archaeologia*, XVIII, 1911.

73 VIGNIER, C., *L'aventureux art Scythe*, Paris.

74 ZAKHAREV, V., 'Sur l'origine de l'art populaire russe', ESA, No. V.

Russian

75 BONDAN, N. N., 'Torgoviye snosheniya Olvii so Skifii v 6–5v', *S.A.* XXIII, 1955.

76 CHVOJKA, V. V., 'Mogili srednyavo Dniepra', *TR AS* XII, L. 1921.

77 EDING, D. N., *Reznaya skulptura Urala*, Moscow, 1940.

78 GORODTSOV, B., 'Dako-Sarmatskie religioznie elementi v Russkom narodnom iskusstve,' *Trud. Gos. Istoricheskovo Muzeya*, 1926.

79 GRABAR, I. (Editor), *Istoriya Russkovo Iskusstva*, USSR Academy of Science, Moscow, 1953, Vol. I.

80 GRAKOV, B. D., *Kamenskoe gorodishche na Dniepre*, USSR, 1954.

81 GRIAZNOV, M. P., *Pervii pazirsky Kurgan*, Leningrad, 1950.

82 KISELEV, S. V., *Drevnaya istoria ujnoi Sibiri*, USSR Academy of Science, Moscow, 1951.

83 KOZLOV, P. K., *Kratkie otcheti ekspeditzii po issledovanii severnoi Mongolii* Leningrad, 1925.

84 MELIKOVA, A. A., *K voprosu pamiatnikov skifskoi kulturi na territorii srednei Europi*, S.A. No. 22, 1955.

85 MELIKOVA, A. A., *Razkopki pamiatnikov Skifskovo vremeni v Moldavii.*

86 MESTCHANINOV, J. J., 'The value of linguistic material in a study of ancient monuments (in Russian)', *GAIMK*, No. I, 1932.

87 MONGAIT, A. L., *Arkheologia v SSSR*, Moscow, 1955.

88 NIKORADZE, G. K., 'O nekotorom snachenii Zemo-Avchalskoi Mogili' *RANION, Institut Arkheologii i iskustvoznaniya, Trudi sektzii arkheologii*, Moscow, 1928.

89 PIOTROVSKI, B. B., 'Razvitie Skotovodstva v Zakavkazie', *SA*, XXIII, 1955.

90 POGREBOVA, N. N., 'Raboti Skifskoi stepnoi ekspeditzii na Nijnem Dniepre', *Kratkie soobshcheniya Instituta Arkheologii 4*, Kiev, 1955.

91 RAVDONIKAS, V., *Naskalniya izobrajeniya Belovo Moria*, Moscow, 1938.

92 RUDENKO, S. I., 'Skifskaya problema i Altaiskia nahodki', *Izvestia AN SSSR*. Seria istorii i filosofii, 1944, No. 6.

93 *Drevnaya kultura Beringovo Moria, Eskimosskaya problema*, 1947.

94 *Kulturnóe naselenie gornovo Altaya v Skifskoe vremia*, USSR Academy of Science, Moscow, 1953.

The Scythians

95 SMIRNOV, G. D., 'Skifskoe gorodishche i selishche "Bolshaya Zaharka",' *KSIIMK*, 1949.

96 SPITZIN, A. A., *Kurgani Skifov-paharei, IAK*, Petrograd, 1916.

97 TARASSUK, S. I., *Imena skifskich tsarei na monetach iz Dobrudji, KSIIMK*, No. 63, 1956, USSR Academy of Science.

98 TSALKIN, K., *K izucheniu loshadei iz kurganov Altaia, MIA*, Moscow, 1952.

99 VITT, V. O., 'Loshadi Pazirskich kurganov', *S.A.* 16, 1952.

100 *Voprosi Skifo-Sarmatskoi arkheologii*, USSR Academy of Science, 1952.

101 ZAKHAROV, A. A., 'Dve Egipetskiya statuetki naidenniya v zapadnoi Sibiri', *RANION, IV Sektzia arkheologii i iskustvoznaniya*.

102 ZELENIN, D. K., *Kultura Angonov v Sibiri*, ML, 1936.

Hungarian

103 GÉZA NAGY, *Néprajzi Füsetek*, No. 3, Budapest, 1895.

Sources of Illustrations

Original photographs for the plates were supplied by the Hermitage Museum, 1, 3, 5, 6, 9, 10, 14, 15, 19–23, 26, 29, 30, 32–4, 38–40, 59; Society for Cultural Relations with the U.S.S.R., 2, 7, 8, 11, 12, 17, 24, 35–7, 48, 57, 58; Victoria and Albert Museum (Crown copyright), 4, 13, 27; Ashmolean Museum, 16, 18, 41, 44, 49, 50; British Museum, 31, 45, 51, 52, 56, 61, 62; John Freeman, 53, 55; Universitets Old-saksamling, Oslo, 42, 43; Guildhall, London, 54; Edwin Smith, 60.

Figures 22, 23, 53 are reproduced from M. Rostovtzeff's 'Iranians and Greeks in South Russia' by courtesy of the Oxford University Press. Figures 3, 12, 14, 19, 48, 49, 51, 52 B.M., are reproduced from E. Minn's 'Scythians and Greeks' by courtesy of the Cambridge University Press. The drawings for figures 7, 11, 13, 15–18, 30, 61, 66–69, are by Mrs. Scott. The maps, figures 2, 20, 24 are by Mrs. G. E. Daniel and figure 50 by J. Woodcock after Bondar, Sovetskaya Arkeologia XXIII, 1955, p. 58. All the objects are preserved in the Hermitage Museum, Leningrad, unless otherwise stated.

The poem on page 122 is reproduced by courtesy of Constable and Co.

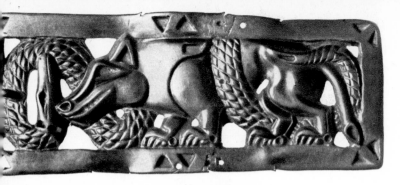

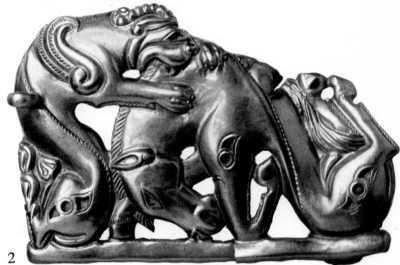

2

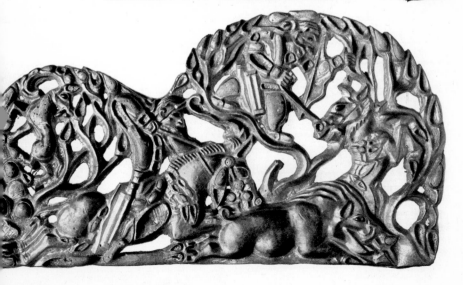

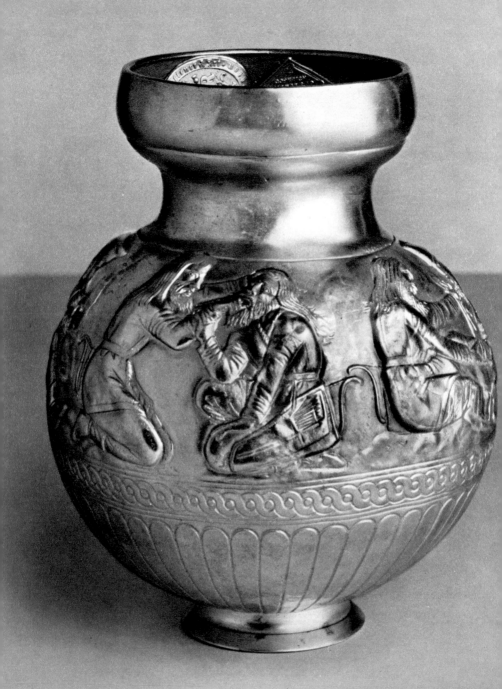

4

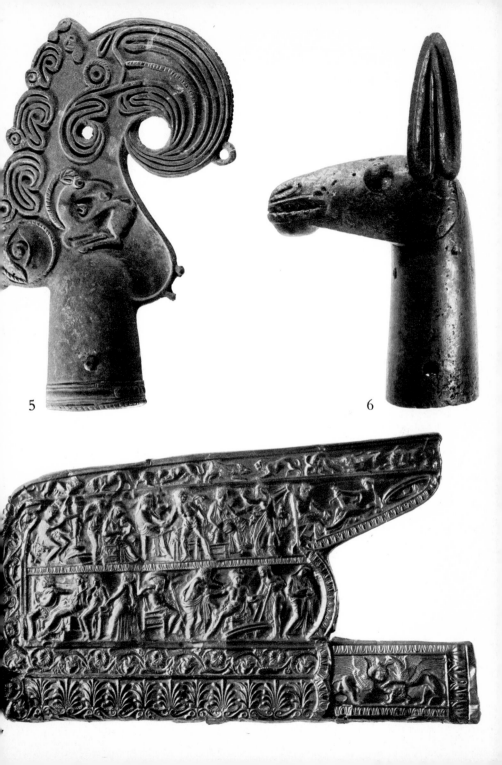

5

6

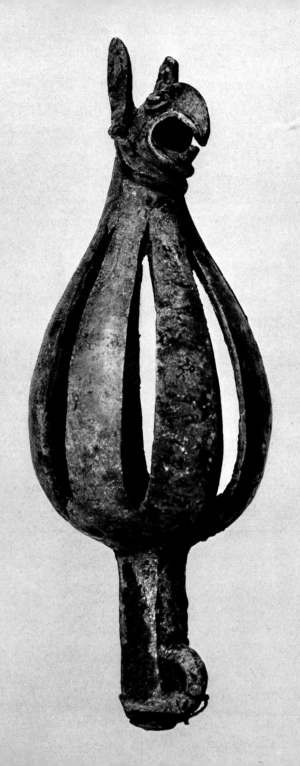

8

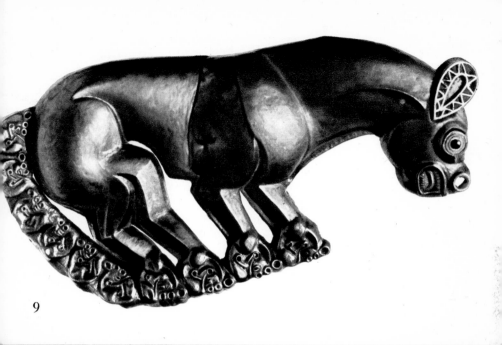

9

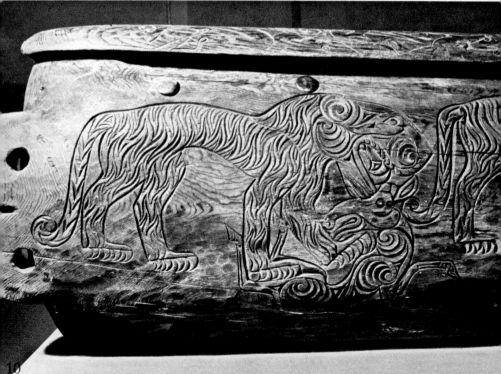

10

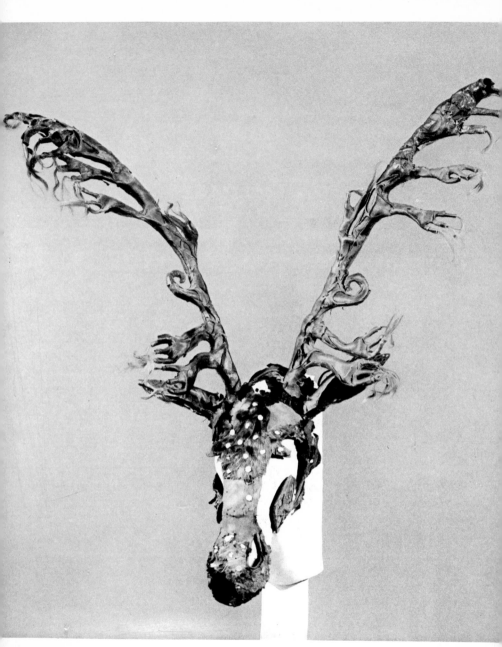

11

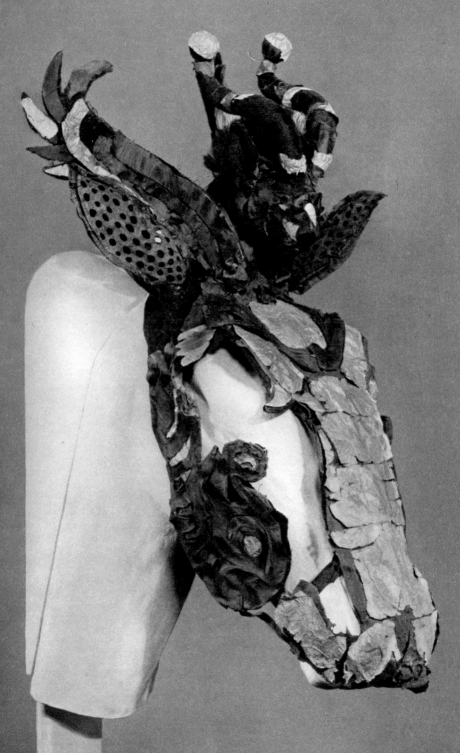

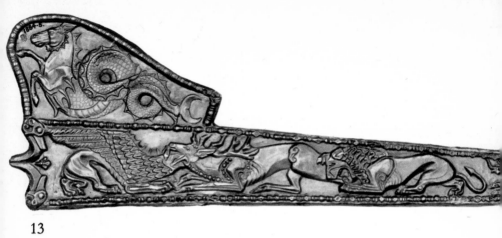

13

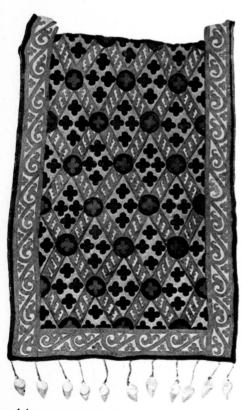

14

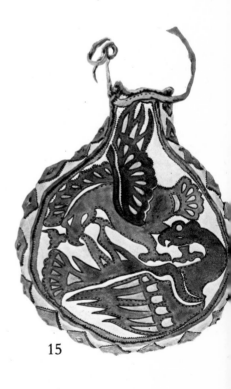

15

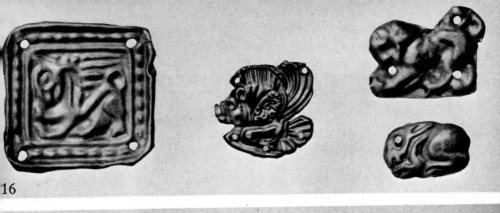

16

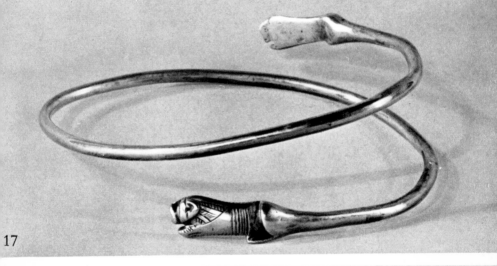

17

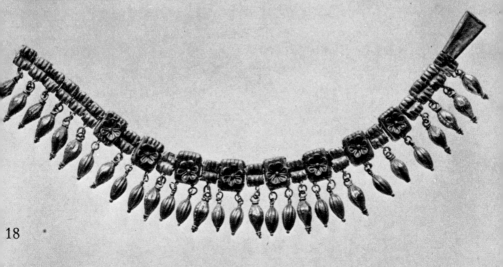

18

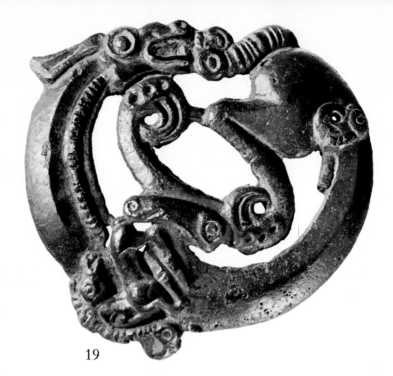

19

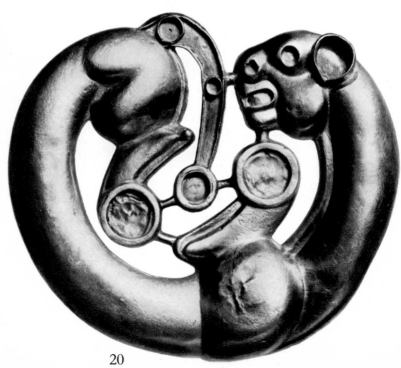

20

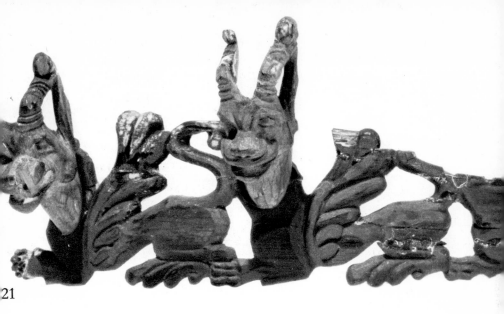

21

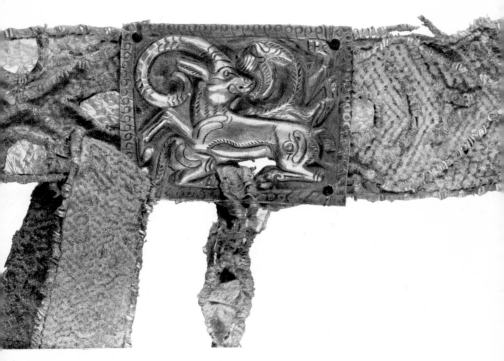

22

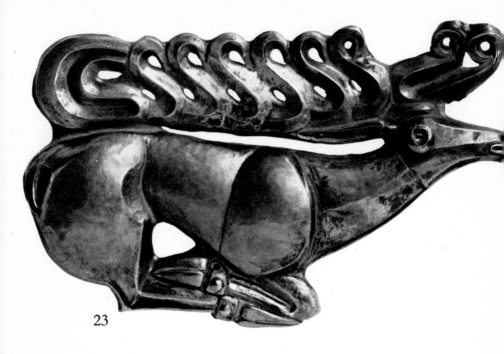

23

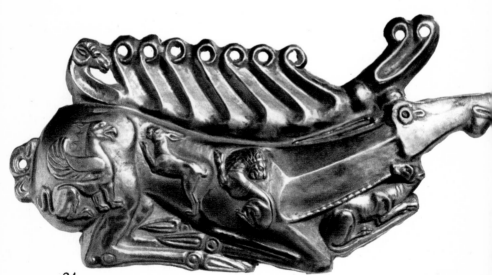

24

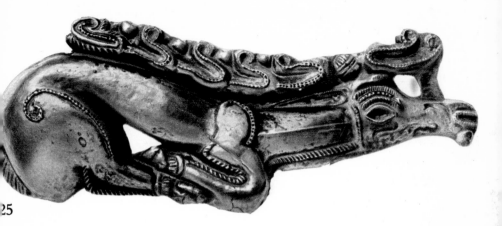

25

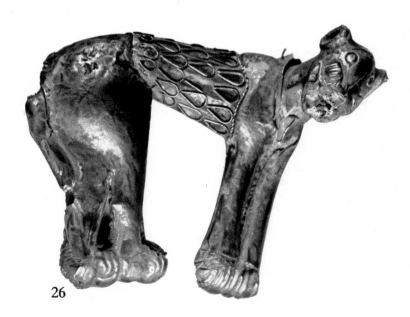

26

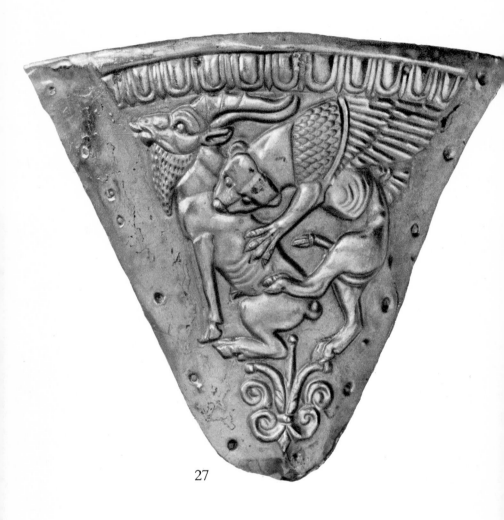

27

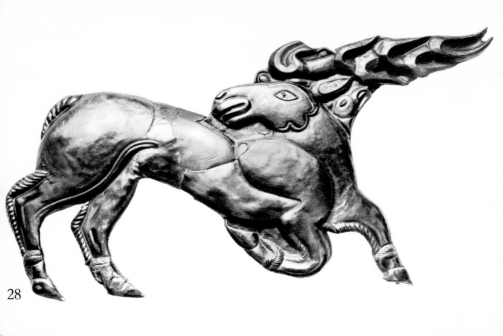

28

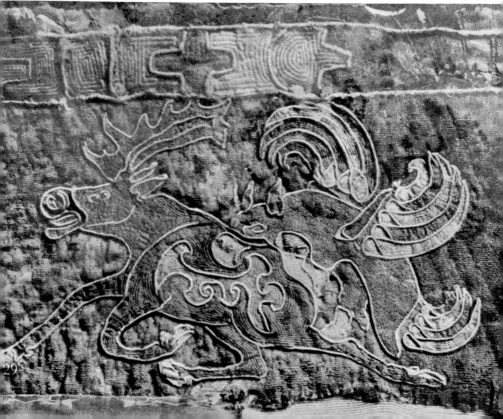

29

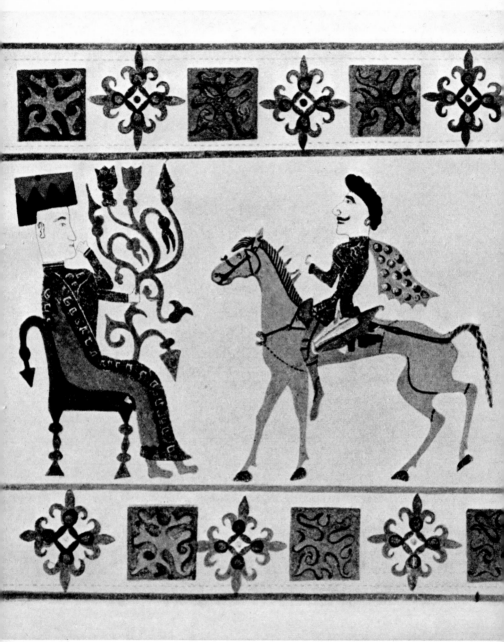

30

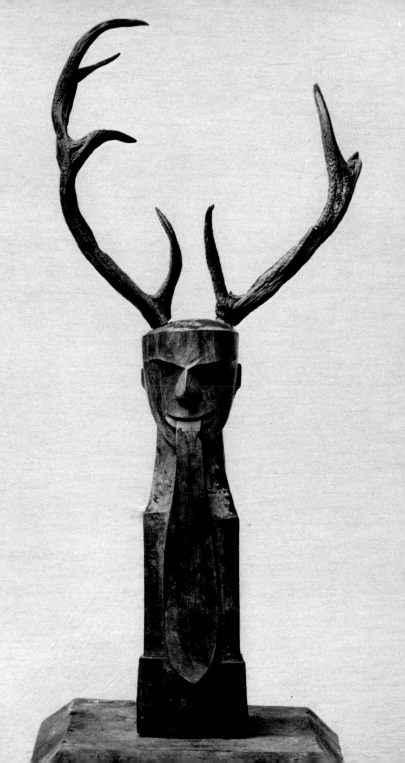

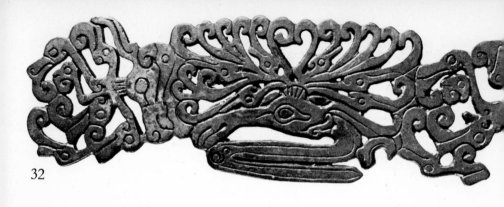

32

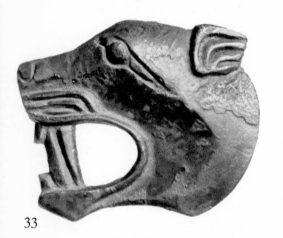

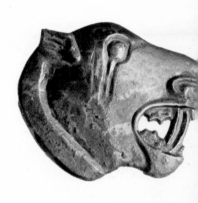

33

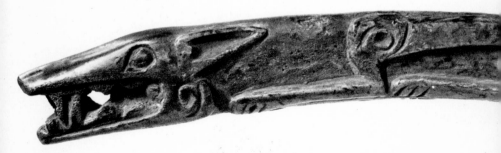

34

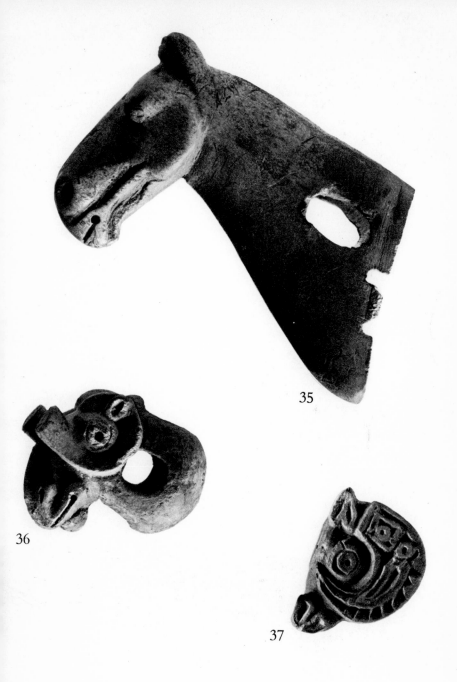

35

36

37

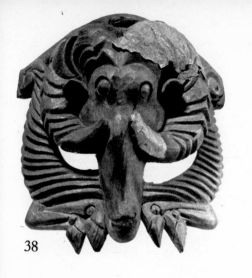

38

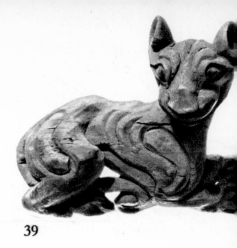

39

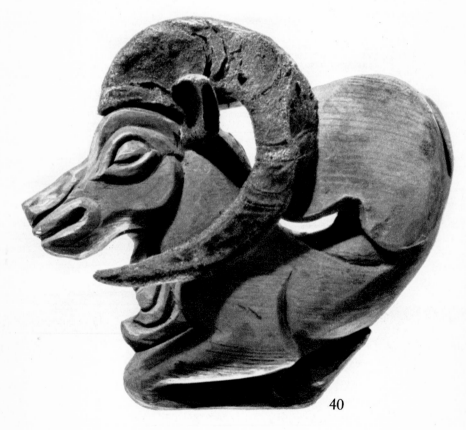

40

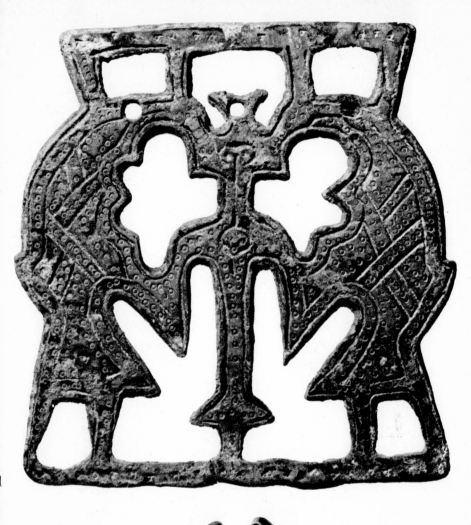

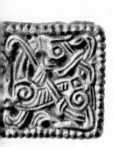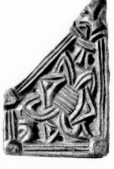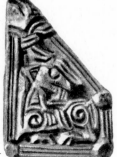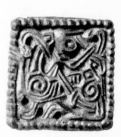

2

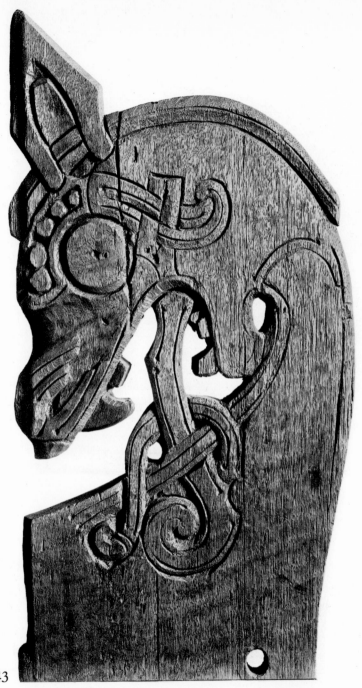

43

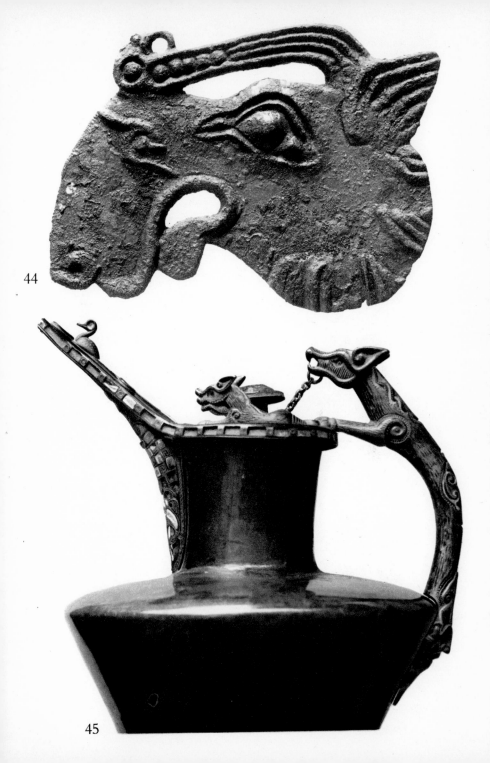

44

45

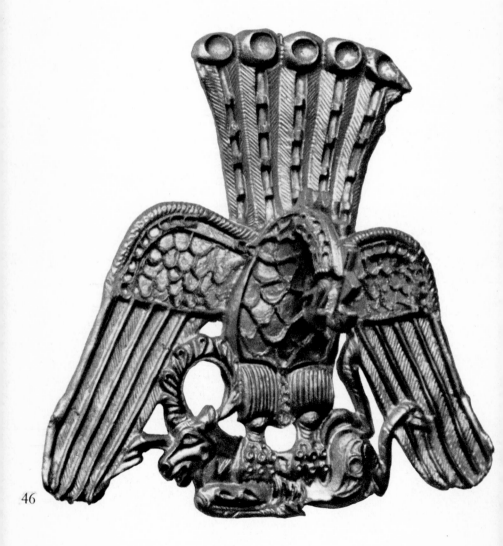

46

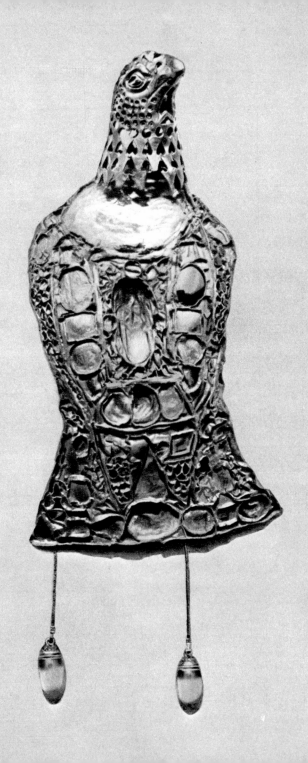

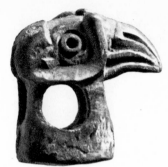

48

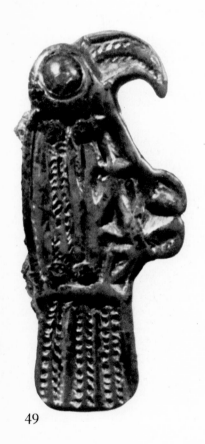

49

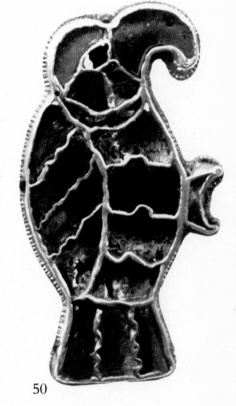

50

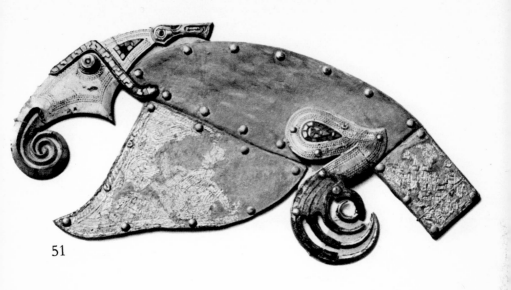

51

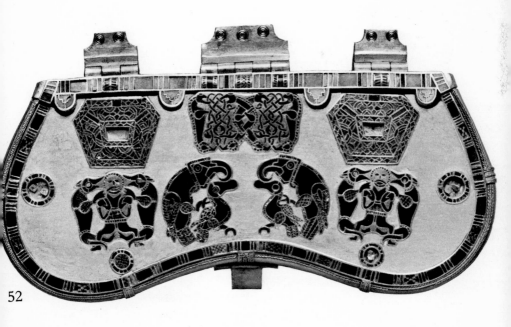

52

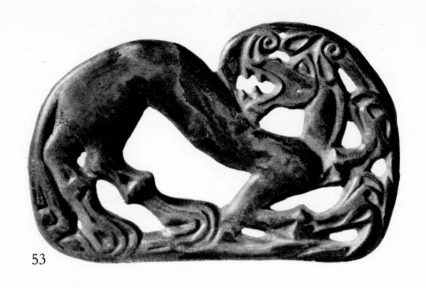

53

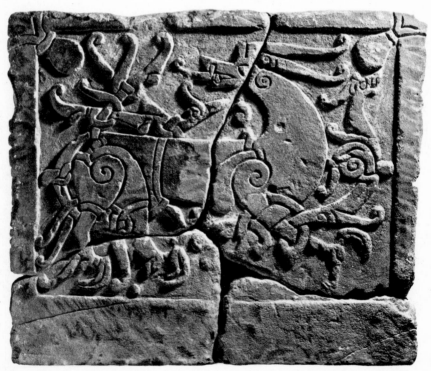

54

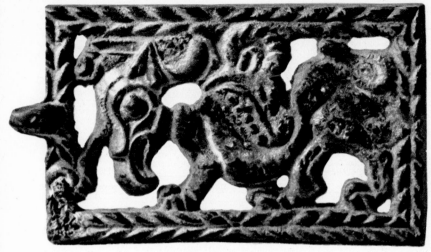

55

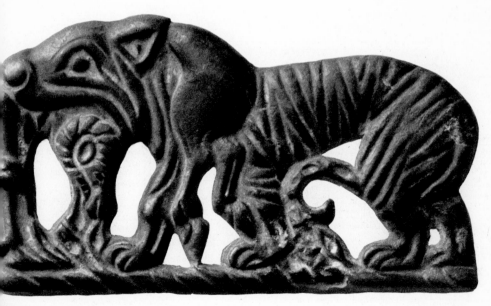

56

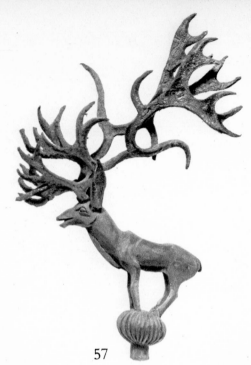

57

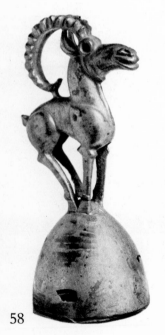

58

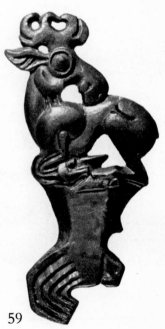

59

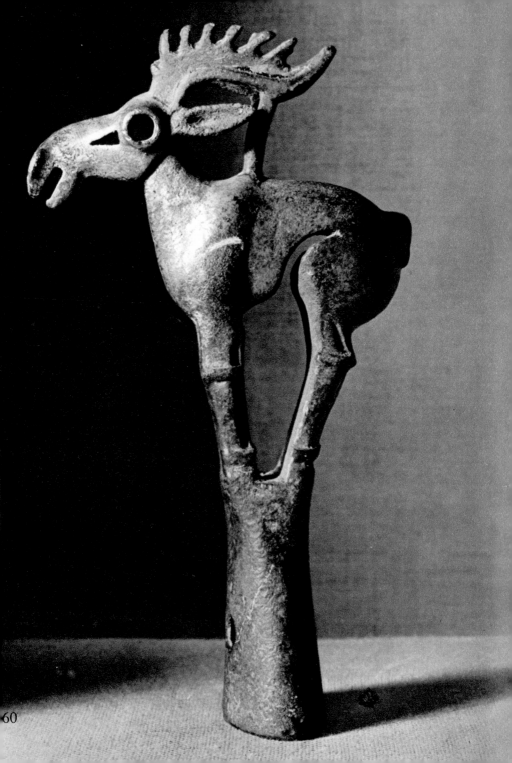

60

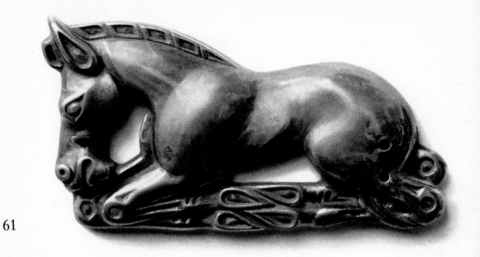

61

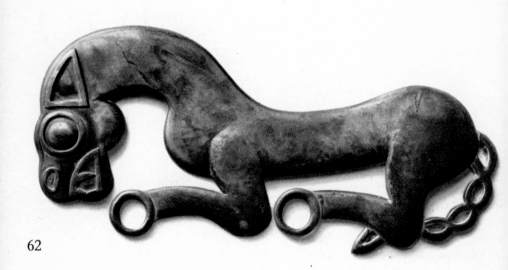

62

Notes on the Plates

1 An imaginary beast, possibly a wolf, and a serpent locked in combat. A gold plaque from Siberia, originally adorned with stone and paste inlay. Indefinite date. Hermitage Museum.

2 A horse being attacked by a lion. One of a pair of cast gold belt buckles from Peter the Great's Siberian collection, now preserved in the Hermi∕tage Museum. About 4½ in. wide. Date indefinite.

3 The Hunt. A Siberian belt buckle in the shape of a horizontal B. Pierced gold. III∕II c. B.C. Hermitage Museum.

4 Electrum vase of Greek workmanship from Kul Oba, near Kerch. IV∕III c. B.C., 5½ in. high. The original is in the Hermitage Museum. This photograph is of an electrotype in the Victoria and Albert Museum. Crown copyright.

5 Cast bronze standard in the shape of a bird's head, from Mound 2 at Ulski in the Kuban. About 11 in. high. VII∕VI c. B.C. Hermitage Museum.

6 Cast bronze pole top in the shape of a mule's head from Kelermes in the Kuban. About 8 in. high. VII∕VI c. B.C. Hermitage Museum.

7 Gold gorytus casing of Ionian workmanship from Chertomlyk, south Russia. About 18 in. long and 12 in. high. IV c. B.C. According to C. Roberts (*Archäol. Anzeiger*, 1889, p. 151) the scene probably represents Achilles on Skyros among the daughters of Lycomedes, inspiration for it having been found in an earlier work by Polygnotus. Hermitage Museum.

8 Cast and hammered bronze rattle in the shape of a bird from Kelermes in the Kuban. About 12 in. high. VII∕VI c. B.C. Hermitage Museum.

O

9 A chased gold leopard decorated with amber and enamel inlay from Kelermes in the Kuban. Possibly the centre-piece from a round shield. Length, about 12 in. VII-VI c. B.C. Hermitage Museum.

10 Detail of a wooden coffin from Başadar in Siberia. VI-IV c. B.C. Hermitage Museum.

11 Antler-crowned horse's head-dress in felt, leather, copper and gilt hair, from Mound 1 Pazirik, eastern Altai. Second half of V c. B.C. Hermitage Museum.

12 A horse's head-dress surmounted with the head of a horned, lion-griffin, constructed of felt, leather, copper and gilt hair, from Mound 1, Pazirik eastern Altai. Second half of V c. B.C. Hermitage Museum.

13 Gold casing on a swordsheath from Kul Oba, Crimea, with the Greek inscription ΠΟΡΝΑΤΟ. 27 in. long. Mid-IV c. B.C. The original is in the Hermitage Museum. This photograph is of an electrotype in the Victoria and Albert Museum. Crown copyright.

14 Felt saddle-cloth from Mound 5, Pazirik, eastern Altai. The crosses may symbolize the sun. Mid-V c. B.C. Hermitage Museum.

15 Leather flagon with appliqué patterns from Mound 2, Pazirik, eastern Altai. About 5 in. high. Second half of V c. B.C. Hermitage Museum.

16 Gold costume trimmings from Mound 2 at Kerch, Crimea. Twice their original size. V-IV c. B.C. Ashmolean Museum.

17 Gold neck circlet with lion terminals from Chertomlyk, south Russia. IV c. B.C. Hermitage Museum.

18 Gold necklace from Mound 3 at Kerch, Crimea. V-IV c. B.C. Ashmolean Museum.

19 Cast bronze circular ornament in the form of a contorted animal. Found near Simferopol, Crimea. VII-VI c. B.C. Hermitage Museum.

20 A cast gold ornament of a panther twisted into a circle. The eye, nostril, ear, claws and tail were originally filled with inlay. From Peter the Great's collection, now in the Hermitage Museum.

21 Carved wood neck circlet from Mound 2, Pazirik, eastern Altai. Second half of V c. B.C. Hermitage Museum.

22 Fragment of a belt with its silver buckle still in place from Mound 2, Pazirik, eastern Altai. Second half of V c. B.C. Hermitage Museum.

23 Chased gold stag, probably the centre-piece of a shield, from Kostrom-skaya in the Kuban. About 12 in. long. VII-VI c. B.C. Hermitage Museum.

24 Gold stag of Greek workmanship, probably the centre-piece of a shield, from Kul Oba, Crimea. About 12 in. long. IV, possibly V c. B.C. Inscribed ΓΑΙ Hermitage Museum.

25 Gold stag, probably the centre-piece of a shield, from Tapioszent-marton, Hungary. The eye and ear were originally filled with inlay. Not later than early V c. B.C. Budapest National Museum.

26 Cast bronze figure of a lioness overlaid with gold leaf, the centre of the body formed of gold wire partitions filled with inlay. From Altin Oba, Crimea. V-IV c. B.C. Hermitage Museum.

27 One of a set of four gold ornaments adorning a wooden rhyta from The Seven Brothers Barrow in the Kuban. Height 3½ in. V c. B.C. The original is in the Hermitage Museum. This photograph is of an electrotype in the Victoria and Albert Museum. Crown copyright.

28 Gold Scythian stag, perhaps a fragment from a combat group, from Zoldhalompuszta, Hungary. V-IV c. B.C. National Museum, Buda-pest.

29 Quilted and appliqué-worked scene of a griffin attacking an elk from a large woven wool carpet, of Scytho-Siberian workmanship, found in the grave of a Mongoloid chieftain at Noin Ula, Mongolia. I c. A.D. Hermitage Museum.

30 Detail from a wall-hanging worked in appliqué felts showing a mounted warrior in the presence of the Great Goddess, from Mound 5, Pazirik, eastern Altai. 4½ m. by 6½ m. Last quarter of V c. B.C. Hermitage Museum.

31 Carved wood, antler-crowned head from Ch'ang-sha in the Hunan, China. IV-III c. B.C. British Museum.

32 Bronze belt buckle or horse's frontlet worked with an antler design, from the Kuban. About 6 in. wide. IV c. B.C. Hermitage Museum.

33 Cast bronze ornamental plaques from horse-trappings. A: Lion's head, from the necropolis of Nymphæum at El Tegen, Straits of Kerch, first half of IV c. B.C. Height, 2 in. B: Lion's head, from Chigirin, Dniepr district, south Russia. Height, 2 in. VI-V c. B.C. Hermitage Museum.

34 Bone hilt carving of a wolf, from Abramovka in the Black Mountain district near Orenburg. Uncertain date. Hermitage Museum.

35 Carved bone head of a horse from Kelermes in the Kuban. VII-VI c. B.C. Hermitage Museum.

36 Carved bone head of a ram from Kelermes in the Kuban. VII-VI c. B.C. Hermitage Museum.

37 Carved bone head of a mountain goat from Kelermes in the Kuban. VII-VI c. B.C. Hermitage Museum.

38 Carved wood harness decoration in the form of a head of a mountain goat, from Mound 1, Pazirik, eastern Altai. 4 in. wide. Second half of V c. B.C. Hermitage Museum.

39 Carved wood figure of a cat on a bridle from Mound 4, Pazirik. Last quarter of V c. B.C. Length, 2½ in. Hermitage Museum.

40 Carved wood figure of an ibex from a bridle from Mound 2, Pazirik. Second half of V c. B.C. Length, 2½ in. Hermitage Museum.

41 Bronze horse⁄trapping in the form of the Great Goddess flanked by supporting beasts, from near Amiens, France. Migration period. Ashmolean Museum.

42 Bronze mountings from Borre in Norway. Late Viking period. Uni⁄versitets Oldsaksamling, Oslo.

43 Figure⁄head of a horse from the Gökstadt Viking ship. Late Viking period. Universitets Oldsaksamling, Oslo.

44 Bronze plaque of a horse's head from Kerch, Crimea. V c. B.C. Ashmolean Museum.

45 Bronze handle in the shape of a wolf from a flagon found at Basse⁄Yutz in Lorraine. IV⁄III c. B.C. British Museum.

46 Gold and inlaid eagle, probably a crest from Siberia. Hermitage Museum. This photograph is from an electrotype in the Victoria and Albert Museum. (Crown Copyright.)

47 Gold and inlaid eagle from the Treasure of Petroasa in Romania. Sarmatio⁄Gothic period. IV c. A.D.

48 Carved bone head of a bird from Kelermes. VII⁄VI c. B.C. Hermitage Museum.

49 A bronze bird of V⁄VI c. A.D. Frankish workmanship. 2½ in. high. Ashmolean Museum.

50 A bronze and enamel bird from Picquigny on the Somme. Frankish, V⁄VI c. A.D. 2¾ in. high. From Sir Arthur Evans's collection, now in the Ashmolean Museum.

51 A double-headed gold and enamel bird from the disk fixed to the boss on the shield found at Sutton Hoo, Suffolk. 655-656 A.D. Length, 10 in. British Museum.

52 Gold and enamel purse from Sutton Hoo, Suffolk. 655-656 A.D. Length, 7½ in. British Museum.

53 Bronze ornament in the shape of a horizontal B from the Ordos. IV-I c. B.C. Length, 4 in. British Museum.

54 Saxon slab from old St. Paul's churchyard. Guildhall Museum, London.

55 Bronze harness mount, or perhaps part of a belt buckle from the Ordos. IV-I c. B.C. Length 2½ in. British Museum.

56 A tiger devouring a ram. Ordos bronze. IV-I c. B.C. Length, 3½ in. British Museum.

57 Cast bronze finial in the form of an ibex from Minussinsk, Siberia. Early bronze age. Hermitage Museum.

58 Cast bronze Scythian decoration from a horse-trapping found near Chigirin. VI-V c. B.C. Hermitage Museum.

59 Carved wood finial of a stag adorned with leather antlers from Mound 2, Pazirik. Second half of V c. B.C. Hermitage Museum.

60 Elk pole-finial in bronze. Han dynasty. Height, 7 in. British Museum.

61 Silver appliqué plaque of a mule. Ordos. Length, 6 in. British Museum.

62 Silver appliqué plaque of a tiger. Han dynasty. Length, 6½ in. British Museum.

Index